Living The Danish Way Of HYGGE

The Secrets of a Happy and Healthy Life

Brenda Hannison

Disclaimer

The information contained in "Living the Danish way of HYGGE" is meant to serve as a comprehensive collection of strategies that the author of this eBook has done research about. Summaries, strategies, tips and tricks are only recommendation by the author, and reading this eBook will not guarantee that one's results will exactly mirror the author's results. The author of the eBook has made all reasonable effort to provide current and accurate information for the readers of the eBook. The author and it's associates will not be held liable for any unintentional error or omissions that may be found. The material in the eBook may include information by third parties. Third party materials comprise of opinions expressed by their owners. As such, the author of the eBook does not assume responsibility or liability for any third party material or opinions. Whether because of the progression of the internet, or the unforeseen changes in company policy and editorial submission guidelines, what is stated as fact at the time of this writing may become autdated or inapplicable later.

Table of Contents

TO LIVE AS HYGGE(INTRODUCTION) 1

Peace of mind in the Danish way.......................5

WHAT TO DO TO ACHIEVE A HEALTHY LIFE...................8

The principles of a happy and healthy life.......................11

REFLECTIONS ON HEALTHY LIVING 13

HEALTHY HABITS FOR A HEALTHY LIFE 22

THE SECRET OF A HAPPY AND HEALTHY LIFE...............27

THE SECRET OF A HAPPY AND MOTIVATED LIFE -
SUPPORT YOUR CORE VALUES 31

SECRETS THAT MAKE US HAPPY AND HEALTHY............39

TOP 5 RECOGNIZED TECHNIQUES FOR LEADING A TRULY
HAPPY AND JOYFUL LIFE INDOORS AND OUTDOORS!..60

TRUE FREEDOM - LIVING A LONG AND HEALTHY LIFE..65

HEALTH AND WELLNESS 77

GOLDEN RULES FOR A HEALTHY LIFE...........................90

BUILDING A HAPPY LIFE: 10 MOST IMPORTANT INGREDIENTS.. 97

Live the truth about a happy life 105

THE KEY TO A HAPPY LIFE IS HOW YOU VIEW IT....... 111

ASTROLOGY TO BE HAPPY - HOW TO LIVE A HAPPY LIFE WITH ASTROLOGY 119

THE CORNERSTONE OF LIFE - EVERY HAPPY LIFE DEPENDS ON A PLANNED BASIS 128

TO LIVE AS HYGGE(INTRODUCTION)

Forge t about trying to be "happy as a clam at high water."You can do it better if you are not (for a while) bivalve mollusks, free from the attention of predators. Instead, start thinking, acting and living like a Norwegian.

Why? Because, according to the latest report from a U.N. agency, Norway is the happiest place on earth. Although there is no guarantee that you will still not be desperate, trivialized and trampled, it can help. A reading of the World Happiness Report suggests that it is worth trying.You could probably be a happier person if you just wanted to be Danish, Icelandic, Swiss or Finnish, the next happiest people in the world after the Norwegians. But why settle for less than # 1?

Norway is # 1

What makes the Norwegians so happy? The first thing you need to know is that there is no magic ball of happiness - many things must come together to create a climate of happiness that breaks through the clouds of gloom and melancholy. The U.N. report added great importance to Norway's astonishing economic strength, social support, life expectancy, freedom, generosity and low levels of crime, corruption, and constipation. (Consider the latter as an interpretative reading between the rules of report variables.) No mention was made of triathlons, participation in national wellness conferences, subscriptions to AWR, compliance with the principles in my book (co-author of Grant Donovan) with the title "The Wellness Orgasm" or your ability to recite messages from Robert Green Ingersoll.

I was intrigued by the fact that a full chapter was given in the U.N. report to "restore American happiness." I did not realize that happiness in America needed recovery, at least not until the national accident that occurred on Tuesday, November 8, last year. However, the proposals offered are certainly in order now, and I recommend them all, especially those who may be able to reverse our unusual inequalities, political corruption, division, isolation and distrust at all levels within the borders. I say "within the framework" because, in my humble opinion, the current government has done little to nothing to gain trust.

Individuals in America cannot do much about the above-mentioned system-wide disruptions, but people can influence their destiny in other ways. For example, consider the following changes to increase the outlook for at least some happiness:

Search for white-collar jobs, but settle for each color job instead of none.

Find well-paid jobs.

If you are stuck in a job that pays poorly, then comfort yourself in the report's findings that "an extra $ 100 salary is worth much more for someone at the bottom of the income distribution than someone who already earns much more."

Leave all hope of happiness by "gaining more power over the world." It has been shown that this is not effective in making people 'happier and happier with life'. Throughout thousands of years, people "have gained enormous power all over the world, but it does not seem that people are considerably more satisfied than in the Stone Age." (Don't ask me how they know.)

Focus on coziness and relaxation. The Nordic countries have consistently dominated the top positions in research for five consecutive years; the Danish concept "Hygge" (coziness and relaxation) seems to be a key factor in this success.

REAL wellness comparisons for happiness

Readers of the great daily feature called "A-Word-A-Day" have recently posted happiness-related comparisons; a few may be of particular interest given the U.N. report.

Comparison for calculating the total family happiness of Ted Palomaki: If F is the total family happiness, $F = 0.1H + K + 10W$. H = happiness of man, K = happiness of children and W = happiness of woman.Comparison for calculating a happy marriage by Daniel Fisher: Happy woman = happy life.

Comparison for calculating happiness in old age by Michael Smout: If A is happiness in old age, then $A = X + Y + Z$, where X is someone to talk to, Y is something to do and Z is something to look forward to.Grant Donovan, happiness wellness expert and polymath orator, whom I will present a session on happiness at the upcoming NWC in June, calculated the following formula, which he called "The Ardell happiness comparison":

$H = F + C + EE + M + WM.$

This means that luck follows when these elements marked by the letter symbols are present. Specifically,

F = has the mental freedom to think and say something, C = has the rational ability to think critically and to question everything, EE = eats well and exercises generously, M = embraces the inherent meaninglessness of your life and WM = Experience multiple wellness orgasms daily.

Peace of mind in the Danish way

Who would think the Danes have a secret that we can all appreciate? The Danes seem to be the happiest people in the world. So what's their secret?

In North America, we seem to be squeezed to the brim. We hurry, work too much, do not sleep well, overload and feel miserable. We work excessively so that we can buy too much and spend too much. The result is that we are unhappy, unhealthy and die younger than ever.

So what we have to do is take a step back from the so-called rat race, where the only person who seems to be happiest is the one who somehow stopped all this nonsense and stopped smelling.

Roses at least once a day. But we usually categorize such people as lazy or anything negative.

So what can Danes teach us about happiness? I think they can teach us a lot. In this article, I will explore several ways we can try a few simple habits that make us happier and healthier.

1. Take time to rest and relax several times a day - once in the middle of the day, once in the late afternoon and once in the evening. Do not use text or other technologies while resting. Don't watch TV. Sit back and relax with a cup of tea or coffee.

2. Perform a simple meditation several times a day, preferably in the morning and evening. If you could do it in the afternoon, the better. Meditation does not have to be complicated. It can be as simple as sitting in

a comfortable chair, breathing deeply several times, setting the timer for ten minutes, closing your eyes and concentrating on your breathing. When you hear a buzzer signaling the end of your ten minutes, slowly open your eyes and feel a few seconds how good it is to relax. You can then continue with normal activities.

3. Live as much as possible right now. Do not try to consider the situation or aspects of your day. Instead, try to focus your breathing several times a day. Take the time and enjoy the view everywhere. There is always something beautiful about us. All we have to do is look and see.

4. Village with nature. It can be a simple walk in the park or just go out during the lunch break and find a peaceful green environment. This can restore your energy and help you feel more relaxed. It can also help you focus and live in that moment, not the past or the future.

Performing these steps will give you more peace of mind. This can help you feel healthier and happier. And when the weekend comes, you can practice some of these tips. It will restore your peace and balance.

WHAT TO DO TO ACHIEVE A HEALTHY LIFE

Everyone knows that "health is better than wealth." In today's world, most of us are educated and some of us read a lot. Health information is all around us and easily accessible to people seeking a deeper understanding. They are also free, as much information can be easily found on the Internet, public libraries and hospitals. For those who can afford to buy, all healthcare books are readily available in bookstores.

But with this enormous available knowledge, what have we done? Most of us just read on, and although we may recognize the health benefits of following a healthy lifestyle and the consequences of not following it, most of us tend to discourage it. We always have reasons or apologies to postpone changing our current unhealthy lifestyle until tomorrow. We keep saying that we will certainly follow a healthy lifestyle tomorrow. Tomorrow will be today, and we will leave tomorrow, and it will be forever waiting for tomorrow.

Some of us may even be troubled by minor or non-life-threatening health problems, but we continue to repeat the cycle of late nights, some sleep, drinking, smoking and eating our favorite tasty foods full of unhealthy fats, oil, salt, sugar, colorings, and preservatives. The most important activities are spent at home behind the TV or computer, rattling chocolate bars or crispy chips accompanied by sweetened or alcoholic drinks. Exercise is the furthest in your head. The same applies to eat a lot of fruit and vegetables. Even if you suffer from minor illnesses and poor health, it is still not important to look for medicines and follow a healthy diet. Only the fact that it is not life-threatening, the motivation and energy to change is still not there. We still want to enjoy life to the full, and today's lifestyle is much more attractive than laying the foundation for future health or work to alleviate illness.

Admittedly, living a healthy lifestyle is not easy and requires a huge amount of discipline, but the benefits and value that you get far outweigh the time and effort you put in and are worth every sacrifice you have to make.

You could argue that some people who strive to adhere to a tried and tested regime are still unhealthy. Yes, that's right. There are important factors that can sabotage our efforts to live a healthy life, and these are our hormones and genes. But if we are determined not to give up the fight, miracles through natural healing, professionally prescribed drugs or proven supplements can overcome the odds.

Health can never be taken for granted. We have to work hard to achieve and maintain good health, whatever it takes. Let us not wait to discover too late that life is no longer meaningful or, in the worst case, suffers from long-term pain and torture.

Take care of your health right now. Exercise regularly, eat plenty of fruits and vegetables, eat a healthy diet - low in fat, low in sugar, high in fiber, high in calcium, etc. Keep trimming, work and private life, manage stress effectively, sleep early and drink plenty of water. Our body has natural healing powers. Learn more about natural healing. Learn how to use food as our medicine. If you are already experiencing minor illnesses, you can learn the right type of natural healing procedures or enjoy the right healthy recipes for the right illnesses. Available natural treatments are aromatherapy, floral products, home-made products, juice recipes, etc. Healthy recipes range from lifetime recipes from 5 known world villages, diabetes, allergy-free recipes, fiber-rich recipes and much more. Try to improve your health or treat yourself naturally and holistically to prevent possible side effects or chemical reactions caused by drugs or surgery. You have nothing to lose by trying it before you go the more drastic way. Take good care of your health. Your health is in your hands.

The principles of a happy and healthy life

It was based on a survey of 50 people over the age of 95 and asked, "What would you do differently if you lived again?" Three common themes emerged in the study.

- They want to reflect more.
- They would be more at risk.
- They would do more things that would live on.

I can see how living according to these three principles would lead to a better and more fulfilling life. You can probably figure out how they can apply to your own life if you take the time to consider them.

One of the things I am interested in as a doctor, writer and speaker are how the principles of a good life apply to the concept of a healthy life. Like the people interviewed in the study, I am 95 or 100 years old, and

I suspect many of you do the same. Many of my patients older than 65 often add that they don't want to live that long unless they are healthy. I just assumed that everyone would want to be 100 years old, but my wider patients remind me that being old, sick and vulnerable is not worth living.

REFLECTIONS ON HEALTHY LIVING

With that in mind, how can we apply these three principles to a good life to enjoy health at the age of 95? The first step is to think more about health. Take a few minutes at the beginning and end of each day to think about what you can do to be healthier. You can also think about what you have done earlier in the day to improve your health. What worked well for you? What can you improve? What should you perhaps learn to be healthy?

Reflection means more than thinking about ways to improve your health. It also means that you have to stop and enjoy the process of a healthy life. Slow down and enjoy the experience of exercising or eating healthy food. Feel your heart beating as you walk or run the last few meters. Enjoy the taste of perfectly prepared vegetables. Life lives like a series of contemporary moments, so stop and think when they happen.

Second, you need to take a greater risk. Be prepared to overcome your current experience. Take the chance to do something you've always dreamed of but were afraid to try. Imagine what you would do if you knew you couldn't fail. Who would you be? What would you do? Who do you want to know? Where would you go?

The risk of becoming healthy

Risk of improving your health. Join the gym you were considering. Make the improvements you have made to your diet. Try it for 30 days. The risk does not have to be huge and impressive. It can only try something you are afraid of being unable to achieve. You may be worried that you can't stop eating red meat or that you can't maintain a training program, but take the risk and start right now.

Leave a healthy heritage

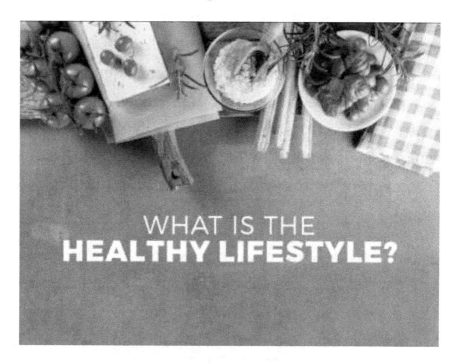

Finally, start doing things that will survive you. Learn to leave a link. Remember that your search for good health will not only affect you. Your decisions, decisions, and actions will affect everyone around you. Your children and grandchildren will learn from you. If they see you exercising and eating healthy, they will do it themselves sooner. If you decide not to eat dessert at work but to eat the salad instead, your colleagues can do the same. We do not live in isolation. We influence and are influenced by the people around us. When you make good decisions and take productive steps around your health, you will have a positive impact on people in your life.

Growth higher by maintaining a healthy lifestyle

Cultivation is the goal of those who want to reach higher heights and look more attractive. This desire to look attractive and beautiful is very basic and innate to all people. Length is a factor that plays a very important role in attracting an attractive personality. Some people suffer from low self-esteem due to the fact that they do not feel charming. The good news for all such people is that height can be increased by gaining the required centimeters as well as maintaining a healthy lifestyle. Yes, it is a fact that higher growth can be easily achieved by pursuing a healthy lifestyle.

You do not have to go to surgery and growth hormones produced in the laboratory, you must rather follow a lifestyle and lifestyle that is healthy and will help you reach higher heights.

Growing up is not just about crazy drugs and pills that increase the slogan of increasing height. They usually do not have positive results. On the other hand, you can maintain a healthy lifestyle and add centimeters to your height. In this respect, some factors need to be considered.

You must always act as a guard dog when choosing food. Health and human growth tend to share a very close relationship and it is the same as trying to achieve the goal of growth. You need to be able to take a type of food and diet that is enriched with all kinds of nutrients, vitamins, and minerals, and it will significantly increase your growth hormones. No junk food is allowed because consumed junk food also consumes stored minerals in the body. So you eat healthily and watch a healthy lifestyle and prolong yourself.

The second that you can add to your healthy lifestyle is exercise routine and exercise. Exercises are considered an integral part of a lifestyle known as healthy. It is a known fact that physical exercises and exercises are much better for health. There are certain exercises in the context of enlargement, such as hanging and stretching, that specifically assist in enlarging immensely.Another important segment of a healthy lifestyle is maintaining the right amount of sleep. If you sleep well for the desired period, it is likely to increase as our growth hormones are activated in our sleep.

So with proper diet selection and regular exercise and exercise, growth hormones are stimulated and these growth hormones are activated when we sleep. Good sleep is, therefore, an essential part of a healthy lifestyle that also counts on prolongation.

Create a healthy life span

In general, life expectancy has increased due to various lifestyle factors

The Center for Disease Control and Prevention offers the following important reasons for our increased life expectancy:

vaccination

- Improving the safety of motor vehicles
- Safety in the workplace

- Better control of infectious diseases
- Determination of cardiovascular death and stroke
- Safe and healthier food
- Healthier mothers and children
- Family planning
- Fluorination of drinking water
- Recognition of the use of tobacco as a health risk

Another factor that contributed to an increase in life expectancy was a drastic reduction in infant mortality.

The biggest part of the expected puzzle that is missing from their list is the ability to stay sick and sick. Modern medicine has been very much involved in the development of methods of masking symptoms, and thus in expanding our ability to live with a condition that has contributed to a longer life span. However, this person still has the cause of the disease or illness. Usually, there are side effects of the treatment with which the patient must live, which is indicated as a mild condition than the original symptom. The question is whether their quality of life is improved when new symptoms of treatment are needed, but rather that the symptoms are being transmitted and changed but not eliminated. This is because the cause has not changed.

Staying healthy is the best quality of life and an anti-aging strategy that can even increase your healthy life expectancy. Imagine that if you were healthy enough to get seriously ill, you would not be involved in taking drugs and drugs that often cause more side effects than the original ones. And once you take these medicines, you probably never get rid of them again, because they don't change anything that supports the real thing.

Do you know why our huge medical resources are not used to stop or prevent the cause?

There is an idea that focuses on the cause and questions about why the disease ever got the body. If the body's immune system is functioning properly, there should be no disease. It is believed that the only way to cope with the disease is that the body is in a certain state that is or should be less than optimal. Standard medical treatments such as medicines, surgery, and chemotherapy help to mask and even alleviate symptoms, but the cause still exists. The surgeon can remove the tumor, but the reason the tumor originally grew is not resolved. Through this medical process, we have come to believe that treating illness or illness is a complicated process that takes time and, of course, a lot of money. Usually, however, it is masking symptoms instead of treating and not restoring well-being.

To look at improving disease and disease prevention, we need to focus on treatment to wellness. The treatment is done when something has happened, wellness prevents it. The focus on wellness can also better serve to heal or improve what has happened than to treat symptoms, because it aims to restore the cause of the desired healthy state, rather than just masking the symptoms.

Studies have shown that the problem is at the cellular level, with body cells designed to perform many functions when they are healthy. Two things work against you. The disease can only thrive in an internal environment that is also not good for your cells. So your body is in a weakened state and the disease is flourishing. Besides, your immune system is weaker and less able to fight this disease. In this state, it is very common for multiple problems to occur at the same time, so the immune system chooses what it is targeting limited options.

Although all of the above areas are important for improving life expectancy, the biggest factor that beats us is still our overall health. If your body is healthy and able to do the job, taking medication every day would not be normal, rather the exception. And many would not spend years with limited lifestyles due to debilitating disorders. The key to the quality of life and life expectancy is to do everything you can to improve your overall well-being.

HEALTHY HABITS FOR
A HEALTHY LIFE

Which way are you going? We are definitely on the way to success! Read on and let's travel together.We all hear people dream of a kind of life where it seems too good to be true. Well, that's not right. Nothing is ever too good to be true. It all depends on how we think and see things. Everything is possible. The only thing that sets us apart from successful people is that we just don't do what is needed. We cannot do anything productive right now and leave it alone the next day. We must have healthy habits for a healthy life. We need consistency and discipline. The secret is simply that we see, learn and study the daily habits of successful people. We have to change our habits and change our lives.

It's so simple!

When we start to change our habits and dedicate and discipline what we do, we will certainly begin to see good positive changes. We must accept it!

Whether we work hard or go home ...

Surrender is never an option. We strongly recommend that you do not even think about it. When you think about it, you are distracted immediately! Nothing is easy. Once we do our best daily habits, what we choose and fight for will undoubtedly bear fruit in the future. Explore the daily habits of successful people. Everyone didn't get what they wanted or dreamed about last night. It may seem that they achieved success at night, but they fought day and night, lost sleep, barely ate, and did not stop resting because they had the best daily habits there. They are determined and determined to achieve success no matter what.

Here are some of the healthy habits of a healthy life:

Mindset - NEVER succeed if we don't believe in ourselves. It is simply not possible if we do not believe in ourselves and what we do. It pulls us down and the next thing we know is living the life of a rogue. Start thinking positive now! You will never regret it!

Discipline - As we have said above, we cannot succeed if we are inconsistent. Success is sometimes defined as consistent actions that are carried out daily.

This is certainly true! At night we can't do anything and expect amazing results all year round. We just do productive things consistently. It is a process, not a one-off agreement. Whether we work hard or go home ... do what you need! I'll never forget it. As our favorite mentor, Jim Rohn said: "Discipline is the foundation upon which all success is built. Lack of discipline inevitably leads to failure. "

Learning - learning never stops. We can study school again and again, but learning never ends. Everyone in this world learns, even though we happen to be teachers. Learning is evidence of growth and development. If we do not learn, we certainly will not earn and grow. The best way to do this is to invest the time of your day in reading books, viewing seminars, speaking and understanding people, inaction and studying successful people. Let's study the daily habits of successful people and apply them to our lives. Be attractive! Become the person people want to be with, not the person people want to avoid.

Be happy! - Being happy certainly helps with our success. Why? That's because if we're happy, we attract more people, positive energy and many more results! Stop complaining, annoying, and constantly thinking about bad thoughts about the situation you are in. Instead, let's look at our lives, evaluate them, and be happy with what we have. Other people in this world are not as fortunate as we are. We are definitely in a better position because we have an internet connection and a computer/laptop / mobile device to read this report.

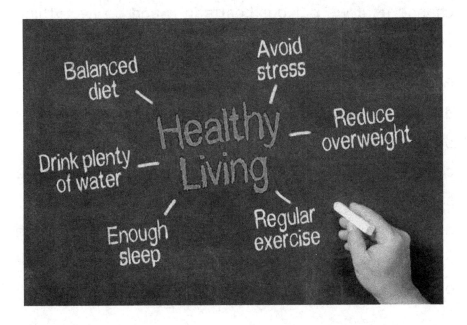

Set your goals - in terms of goals, it must be something we are passionate about and determined to achieve, no matter what obstacles we encounter. Work hard or go home. It depends purely on us, but when I think of my goals, I cannot stop working on myself and my future. Another fantastic proverb from Jim Rohn is "Goals. Nothing will tell you if you let you inspire. There is no one to tell you what you can do if you trust them. happens when you act against them. "Go for it!

Act according to your goals - we keep it simple. It is not enough to wait and expect something to happen. Go outside and let them stand.

These healthy habits for a healthy life will surely change us if we put our hearts in it and do everything we can to make it happen.

Become a go-getter! Go outside and fulfill your dreams! Everything is possible. How do we know? Look outside the world and see how many people have conquered the word "impossible." We can also if we start to see that it is possible. Do what is necessary and feel good. It will certainly pay off in the future. We will soon realize that changing our daily habits will eventually change our lives and who we are.

THE SECRET OF A HAPPY AND HEALTHY LIFE

Life happens; it can be created and destroyed in an instant; all aspects of life, including marriage, success, and defeat. Prepare to land on fire, you may not have another chance.

It was a beautiful June day. I went to the conference, so my husband and I decided to go there and see America instead of flying directly to the destination. The purpose of the conference was to increase my chances of success in my new company.I had the best intention to do it, though I wondered why it would bother me, it didn't work for me. Now I know it wasn't about the conference, but the way.

Many times in my life I have experienced this feeling of separation between what I felt was good for me and what I did to please others. I'm sure you felt the same, including, unfortunately, that you got married. I recently heard the answer to my dilemma; one has to know the meaning of life and go this way.

We drove and talked together, talked about the past, developed our lives, listened to music, just like in movies. Have you ever felt that you are not involved in your life; but instead of watching it and waiting for you to get a big part?

I hear the movies we watch say a lot about our personality. I know that my favorites are musicals, love stories and comedy rocky rocks. Each of the film categories must be happy, educational, must build personality and humanity. I think life is by nature a cluster of happiness. The worst awaits our innate concerns.

Then back to the road; the view and the weather were great. The traffic was stable, no distractions, and I didn't hear about this big bang anywhere else. In a fraction of a second, the car crashed into the concrete partitions on the side of the road that I discovered later. The road was under construction and somehow big orange and white cones led us down instead of creating a safety zone. As I sat or hung inside, I felt pain in my shoulder, I saw a sidewalk under my head over the sunroof; Somehow, with a complete starting point, I waited for the car to go full rotation and land on "hands and feet". Like in movies; staged and planned. I was not afraid; I wasn't panicking. I was calm and waiting for the end of this scene.Everything happened, as I expected, a four-wheeled car, we sat quietly waiting for someone to open the door.

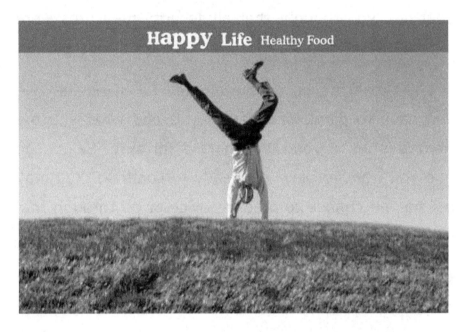

I didn't drive, so when the viewers ran to see if the driver was okay, I got angry, I was as much an actor in this movie as he was; Why wasn't I welcome as it was? I wasn't in the driver's seat. There was no cameraman, only viewers. Everyone followed our next step.

We looked at our husband and smiled. No words, just a smile that confirms a "good shot". I tried to open my side door, it didn't work. The damage to the car was huge. The damage to us was minimal. My husband was hit by a flying object (computer), my elbow was damaged and dripping blood stained my shoes. I wasn't in shock; it was the expected movie scene.We are convinced that you have heard the Big Bang in your life, you thought that all security measures were in place. Think again.

Life is like a movie, you've already taken on the role you have to play. How you play it and what you get from it is up to you. One thing is for sure. Select the role you want to play, get ready to continue. You may not have a chance to practice twice or go through trial and error tactics.

We got a chance to get a general exam without preparation. I stood up with the full understanding that my young approach to life must change. I have to sit in the driver's seat of my own life so things don't happen by accident. No one is here to play a central role in their own lives. It helped me open the door to a new reality that I had to fix things. Random viewers do not want to welcome the event. Listen to your heart; listen to your innate size. You will succeed.

THE SECRET OF A HAPPY AND MOTIVATED LIFE - SUPPORT YOUR CORE VALUES

Core Values and Vision We are talking about dreaming big and achieving meaningful goals by living our core values. When we adapt our decisions and actions to serve these values, we lived inspired and enlightened.Do you serve your core values? If you know your 3 highest values, you can do a simple exercise to see if you deserve your core values.

Let's look at your 3 best values and use "time spent" as a criterion to get an idea of where you are with these values. How much time would you spend on activities that support each of your core values?

Then, based on last week, map how long you spent each of these values.For example, if your top 3 main values are family, work, and health, how much time do you spend watching these top 3 values based on last week?

With "Family Time" we can spend time with our family members, do things together, discuss or share, etc.

"Working time" includes the time you commute, the time you spent at home on your phone or computer, the time you spent outdoors on business trips, etc.

Similarly, you may also decide that the "Health" bucket should include the time spent buying food for your healthy diet, preparing meals, washing dishes, spending time in the gym or using meditation, etc.

Now compare the two-time series and see what trend you see.If you are surprised by the results, what changes do you want to make?

May your core values be your compass. but these values will not appear in your life and are not realized until you make and make similar decisions that support them. Having "love" at the top of the list is a good start. If you do not act or prepare for it, it will quickly take its toll and create guilt. The separation between your value and life will cause stress.

We do not want to go through life in response to every day "urgent" problems and get involved in crisis management. We do not want to live in a stress zone where life is used to responding to what the environment offers us. We want to be in control and live with purpose and joy.

I hope you take the time to complete these exercises. The clearer your values and the more you are willing to serve those values, the more inspired and focused your life. Let your values be your compass for everyday decisions.So you are happy - the secret of finding happiness through spiritual experience

What is the real secret spiritually happy and fulfilled? Why are people who have some form of spiritual basis or religious beliefs happier, healthier and even reportedly living longer than those who do not share the same adaptation with something greater than themselves? Are clairvoyants and the media religious, or is there anything else spiritual? Some of these questions sound familiar? In this Book, we need to quickly and easily look at what I believe to be the real, authentic secret of being happy and also living the life of PASSION, power, and purpose. Interested in more? Keep reading as we take a closer look below. Before I go to the more spiritual elements of this article, I want to share with you what the true SCIENCE of happiness told us. Much research has been done on what creates a happy life ... and the surprising truth is that it is a combination of practicing well-being that nourishes body and mind and causes the soul to smile in and out.

Did you know that the science of happiness can be divided into several simple characteristics? That is true ... and many university studies have demonstrated 6 qualities, including leading to happier, healthier and hopeful people.

- Daily gratitude exercises
- Daily meditation practice
- Healthy food
- Exercise at least 20 minutes each day

A sense of spiritual connection to something greater than ourselves

Last but not least, a belief in a certain purpose in life that gives meaning and strength to what you want to achieve.

Simply put, happiness can be cultivated by maintaining a healthy body (diet and exercise) and, more importantly, by cultivating a healthy mind. Now understand that this is also true. I'm not a religious man. But I believe in the idea that we are all connected and that there is a reason why we live this life together and that we all return to the place of light and love.

From my own experience as a spiritual writer, researcher, and professional publisher, I have learned incredible lessons in life that transformed my sense of myself and my attitude ... from negative and condemning, to blissful, patient and accommodating everyone.For example - Researching near-death experiences for 5 years and interviewing many people who let them convince me that we are ALL connected, that we come from a place of light and love ... and return to the same place when our purpose on this planet is fulfilled.

Exploring the supernatural media for decades has taught me that in each of us there is something timeless and eternal and that every person is filled with soul and spirit that transcends death and continues after the body no longer does it.

This simple realization taught me that nothing is sad.

This happiness and joy is our natural state. That all pain is temporary and all emotions ... even the hard ones, disappear in the light of the mind, which is larger than our body, are here to learn, love and grow ... and one day they will know that every problem that we faced was presented to us as an opportunity for development. This is the secret of true happiness! And it does not come from the belief of dogmas or reading textbooks.

It is the opening of your mind and spirit of power and potential of who and who you are ... and to be grateful for any experience. Take care of your body - take care of your mind and take an adventure.

It ignored the open secret of a healthier and longer life

Most of the food we eat looks very tasty. It is the way food looks and deceives us by believing that it can promote good health. No matter how good the food tastes or how attractive it looks. What matters is the value of the food in it. However, the value of food is destroyed by processing, depletion of nutrients in the soil, use of preservatives, pesticides, etc. When we eat such food, we are exposed to a large number of dangerous degenerative diseases.

The unbalanced nature of the food that people eat today causes overweight. This is because food contains more calories than better food value. Add-ons can correct this imbalance. To prolong the shelf life of some processed foods, radiation is used to kill microorganisms. However, this process destroys important nutrients such as fat-soluble vitamins and antioxidants.

Therefore, it is necessary to use accessories. It is denatured during food processing. The food is refined and removes all life poisoning. These are bran, which is filled with minerals and vitamins. When buying vitamin B pay attention to the color ... bran.

The temperature to which the food is exposed also contributes to the depletion of vital nutrients. Therefore, you must replenish your supplement's inventory. We live in critical times. The hardships in life cause stress. It is this stress that produces hormones that bombard your body's cells 10,000 times a day. Cell, Ex. Day. This will cause your cells to run out, so you look much older. The use of supplements, especially antioxidants, may reduce this effect. It is estimated that 6 billion pounds of chemicals are thrown into the environment each year. Air, water, and soil are affected. Plants that grow in such soils absorb these toxins, which eventually reach our bodies.

Unless you have detoxifying nutrients, dangerous diseases become the order of the day. Vitamin C is a nutrient that detoxifies the human body. You can get vitamin C from some supplements. Our lifestyle may also require the use of accessories. The smoker destroys the reserves of his vitamin C. Alcohol also plays a role in diet depletion.

We recommend using accessories. Many diseases can be prevented by maintaining a balanced diet. Treating food, using preservatives and radiation, lifestyle and stressful life are some of the ways the body is focused on nutritional supplements. If we respond positively to this demand, our lives can be long, happy and healthy.

SECRETS THAT MAKE US HAPPY AND HEALTHY

We all want to be happy and happy and do everything we can to be. Unknown secrets and happy events change and affect our lives in many ways. Incomplete events can change our situation. "Little" secrets in life can keep us healthy and we don't have to focus on heaven to make our life happier and busier. Your doctor's pure clique about your health, your partner will show you his true love for you, a true friend who cares about you and many other such happy moments can stimulate your life.

Good health, disease-free life, choice of different options, good food can bring joy to our sad life. A true friendship, an upcoming man, a successful career can give you a positive and enthusiastic feeling of life in general. When you realize that somebody makes you feel good. Happiness is what you are always looking for.

What makes you happy and healthy?

A real friendship. It can do wonders. Everyone wants a

loyal friend they can trust. He must be able to share all fears, fears, and feelings without reservations. A reliable person who is there when you need him. True friendship cannot be purchased. It must be cultivated during a certain period

Life without the disease. Everyone wants to be fixed and fixed. If the doctor gives clean shit, you will feel relieved. "Health is prosperity". When you are in good condition, you will be happy. It is a blessing in disguise, we bless good health

Have more choices in life. People like more preferences and fulfill their desires in a way that suits them best. Diverse decisions allow a person to choose the best option.

A spouse. Knowing that your partner loves you very much can make you very happy. A successful marriage is what they hope for. An understanding and caring partner that you can trust can make a big difference in your married life

A stress-free life. A trouble-free life can do wonders for someone's character. One can be more relaxed, cheerful and take life as it comes. He or she can lead an interesting and exciting life and not be confronted

with problems today

Financial security also makes you feel comfortable. The basic needs must be met. Everything that needs to be earned must be enjoyed. Everyone works hard to reach both sides and wants to earn more to make life easier and more comfortable.

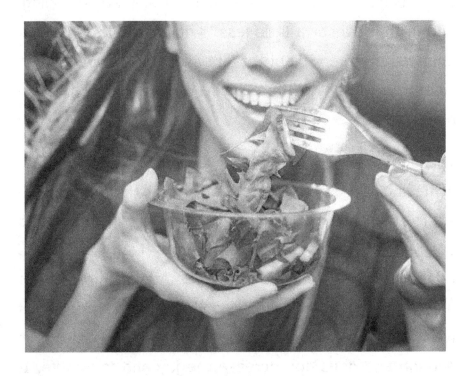

When a man can provide his family with all the conveniences of daily life, he feels happy. If he earns more and is successful in his career, it requires a party

Happiness is a state of mind. But a person's circumstances must also be conducive to making someone feel that life is worth living. He or she strives to be successful in leading a blissful life.

The secret to creating happiness

There are countless books written about finding happiness. Everyone is looking for happiness, whether they realize it. Happiness is a natural state of being, and in that sense, a little less is not normal for people, animals or even plants. A houseplant in the shade when the sun shines in a closed window is not a happy plant.

The good news is that recent research has found that achieving a certain state of well-being and self-sufficiency ensures a comfortable state of comfort and does not have to worry about normal health problems, relationships or financial problems. Adding more is not only unnecessary but does not increase the feeling of well-being or happiness of iota. In other words, it is enough and does not increase the joy and joy of life. It is true in all aspects of earthly life.

Animals have a significant advantage in this respect because they are not connected to intellectual matters such as humans so that they can live their entire lives in what would be considered a natural grace. Animals do not anticipate the future, nor can they remember and care for the past as humans, so you can understand why they have such an advantage in a more direct, intensified and extensive contemporary experience without the complications of ego-identification. Animals and plants have no egos to deal with.

People, on the other hand, have a much more complicated life since birth, sometimes complications of a negative nature. These negative complications can be such as financial problems, health problems, relationship problems, and other psychological problems that animals simply do not have to solve. But people do.

Life is easy if you know how to do it.

By avoiding all the "continuing negative challenges" brought to this life by previous life experiences, the lives you have lived in different times and places, for the first time you open your eyes after birth as a really small person, vulnerable and completely dependent on your survival parents, without prior knowledge and experience.

You have likely lived before, and your present life in this physical world is influenced by the nuances of many past experiences with the reincarnated past of the past, probably yourself, souls, qualities and abilities or shortcomings. inheritance from your current parents.

You also (unconsciously) bring to this life all the knowledge and information you have learned over the centuries about your soul/entity. This knowledge is not consciously available for a variety of reasons but can be intuitively portrayed through long inspirational impulses and imagination, as well as in your dream adventures. Often you unwittingly rub your elbows on your likely self, while other characters appear in your dream dramas.

Nothing has ever been lost mentally, and the first peak of knowledge that you have learned in any previous life of any age is preserved as what can be considered in this life as an "instinct" built into your genes, but not known to be intentionally available for practical purposes. The physical brain does not contain this knowledge, the conscious mind does.

Before you are born into your current physical body, you have a history of different life experiences. I have now rejected these cases, as I said, describing people born with what I call negative reincarnation luggage, and brings to this life the unresolved challenges of past lives to address them to the present.

These problems can be solved, treated and rejected, except in cases of persistent disease, malformations, limb deficiency, etc., with which you were born. Every illness you are born with has intentionally created and accepted you as a precondition for this life challenge, and will usually be with you for life, but remember that you have created a challenge to learn how to overcome such difficulties.

Assuming you were born with a healthy body, you were free at least a short time after birth. The human body is a gestalt of consciousness consisting of millions of small forms of consciousness of atoms, molecules, and cells that make up the greater physical components of your physical self, and the physical self has a built-in defense against diseases and diseases.

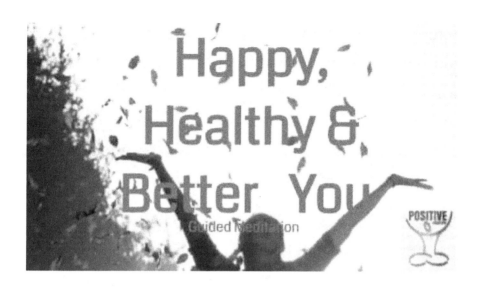

This small cellular consciousness forms what is called "body consciousness." Body consciousness provides a function of unconscious physical activities such as breathing, heart rhythm, and perception. If you were thinking about breathing, you would quickly learn how important body consciousness is. If you thought your heart was beating, you would be in serious stress.

Your cells know what is going on at any given time with every other cell in your body and they make adjustments to correct any imbalances. This corrective capacity is often indicated by the body's immune system. Your body awareness, in collaboration with your self-directed conscious personality, works seamlessly together to create a satisfying life experience.

Cellular collaboration keeps your body so healthy that you don't mentally sabotage the process. The problem is that as a child you begin to learn and accept the beliefs of others almost immediately after birth and that every subjective belief physically influences the child in different ways.

I only mention these things to point out that your body, from the lowest cell to the highest order of intellectual sharpness of the brain, excluding reincarnation baggage, was born perfectly healthy and able to take care of itself.

It is in a natural state of physical balance. You cannot have a full, happy life experience when you are sick.

Wellness is one of the most important conditions for happiness and it is a privilege for all consciousness, including plants and animals. This may sound silly, but people, animals, and plants can also feel a state of happiness, although in different emotional views.

Assuming you had a healthy body at birth and assuming that you have learned nothing and have not accepted harmful beliefs in your life, you would be healthy until you die. Your physical body and personality is a mental creation projected from an inner subjective reality in the three-dimensional physical system (Earth Reality) for a certain period under certain predetermined and predetermined circumstances.

You are what you think you are, no more or less, so you have to think about yourself. I say that you existed before your birth and that you will continue to exist after your death. Awareness is not dependent on a physical body as a condition of existence. Consciousness is eternal, physical bodies are not. You shed physical bodies, just as a snake sheds skin, and when a snake grows new skin, you grow new bodies.

Before you were born, you made relevant decisions that resulted in the body with which you were born; you chose it, it is strengths, and it is a vulnerability for reasons of your design for purposes that only your inner self knows, and you must address it.

I say that your physical self, DE, which you name by your adopted name, was not born in sickness or accident by destiny or a random and unstable god, but is an accurate reflection of a mental process that causes the matter in a perfect reflection of your inner orientation.

You are then what you have made yourself to be. Through mental processes you created the pattern that physical matter assumes, resulting in the physical form that you see in the mirror every day. You are your creator. If you don't like what you have made, you can make adjustments and changes by changing the way you think about yourself. There is no other way.

You cannot blame anyone except yourself for what you are or for your life situation. Neither God nor destiny has led to your present state of being. You are to blame and the good news is that if you are fully responsible for your state of being, you can also change it. Conscious energy is constantly changing and it is your job to drive change more favorably to your satisfaction and fulfillment.

The energy behind the thought, belief, desire, and expectation is propelled into the matter; atoms are collected in a specific physical form, controlled by consciousness. Awareness creates and manipulates substance. Depending on the intensity of these properties, physical substances may disappear rapidly, for example in the incredibly short life of a fruit fly or persistent condition for a very long time, as evidenced by the life of some larger turtles, which sometimes live for hundreds of years.

I'm sorry to have to spend as much time explaining as you expect, but if I didn't, these difficult concepts couldn't be understood for you. I think I went as far as I should, with the background so that I could start on the subject now, good luck.

You have learned from your parents since birth. She perceives the fetus from her womb, sees and hears her mother's belly and then even begins to adapt to her parents' lifestyle. They will learn in a basic way what parents already know. Of course, this learning process continues after birth and is a prerequisite for the child's survival to the early years.

The knowledge the child receives from its parents should never be permanent and the belief that the child has taken it from the parents must be investigated and, if necessary, changed. The parental belief was necessary to survive in the child's early years, but they were not eternal.

This will be a shock to some who read this article, but parents' opinions are not always correct or useful and are certainly not a valid template for structuring life in the neighborhood. To be honest, some children have quite ignorant parents, intellectually confused about the ideal living conditions of life.

I conclude that your beliefs, including those of your parents, can be harmful when it comes to using them as a template to build a happy life. Your life is a reflection of your inner beliefs about yourself, and if your inner beliefs about reality are distorted or reflect negative thoughts and concepts, your life experience will also be distorted and the result will be misfortune.

Here I try to emphasize the importance of "what you believe" in creating a fulfilled and happy personal life. A distorted belief that you do not seem to be in any way linked to the shortcomings you experience in your life, so it can be difficult to associate them with a particular problem in business life.

Imagine that at birth you want a clear, straightforward and effortless journey ahead of you that does not prevent false or distorted beliefs. Imagine negative beliefs such as stones, obstacles or holes, roadblocks on the path of life. At birth, this path is clear and there are few negative opinions, except for those less accepted by your parents. At some point, when you grow up in your youth, you have to explore faith, especially if you have trouble in your life.

Your life is built on the beliefs of existence that you accept from others, such as teachers, clergy, scientists, philosophers, politicians, and medical professionals.

It may seem outrageous, but some of the most harmful beliefs come from religious dogmas related to sin, curse, hell, favorite Satan and Jerry Falwell, "Lake of Fire." The concept of "original sin" or "lagging" can be paralyzing, feeling inadequate or incompetent for people induced by these beliefs.

On TV you have full advertisements from pharmaceutical companies extending the benefits of their miracle cures to keep you healthy, sometimes from diseases, you didn't know existed. Public informational advertisements ask women to inspect their breasts or have a colostomy performed regularly and to prepare for your flu with another almost mandatory vaccination.

Flu shots don't protect you from the flu. Belief in flu shots protects you from the flu.I quote them as examples of how the conviction is convinced of you and is accepted by the process of mental osmosis, without knowing why it unwittingly accepts the advice of others without taking into account its validity. You collect many of your most harmful beliefs without knowing that you are.

Every new belief can be like another albatross hanging around your neck and pushing you down. Most of these beliefs that you unconditionally can begin to include your happiness with distorted, unhealthy beliefs that hinder the free flow of natural universal energy that causes blockages and difficulties in creating a natural, healthy physical reality.

Remember, subjective thoughts, beliefs, desires, and expectations are becoming a reality in the physical world that you experience every day. The external reality is connected from the inner subjective state; subjective becomes objective, the result is a physical reality.

You think it exists and you think you are lucky or suffering. This is your decision; The right to a happy life is your heritage in your world unless you give up your duties.

If you are lazy in investigating your faith, you may have trouble. Which do you think you should stay.It's not that you have to learn anything; it is rather what you have to learn not to do. All you have to do is learn how to open the door so you can keep the natural state of free flow without overcoming it without synchronization. In other words, keep your channels free and unlimited.

Clear your mental paths and reduce obstacles by destroying broken defective or distorted beliefs, and the path to happiness will be ready for new useful beliefs that will flow, and true happiness will replace the old.

In other words, you got a clear path at the beginning of your life, but you started with a dysfunctional mental bag from various sources and saw what happened. Get rid of the mess, get out of the way, and your life will begin to improve almost immediately.

Do not automatically accept what others are telling you, don't trust everything you hear, trust your intuitive knowledge, and you won't be lost. If your life is ruined, you know for sure, your beliefs will be ruined. Faith always comes first, reality follows.

The secret of personal happiness

Here is an oxymoron that blinds me to the idea of happiness and how we can achieve it. Let me start with a general profile of people who have read this book:

- You live in the Western world with all its democratic rights and freedoms.
- You have decent work that deserves an adequate standard of living.
- You have strong personal relationships with family and friends.
- You are married or have ever been.
- You have children.
- You have material luxury: house or apartment, car, clothing, technology (mobile phone, laptop,
- Xbox, etc.).
- You are intelligent, attractive and generally successful in life.
- You had quite a good upbringing from a decent family.
- You follow a hobby or sport you like.
- You are in relatively good health.

This certainly does not apply to anyone reading this article, but I only offer a general overview of the majority of people I think are my readers. Are you surprised how close I got to the truth? Want to know how I discovered it? There are two reasons. Anyone who has materials, democratic freedom, a successful career, friends and family and financial stability, and also has the opportunity and time to think whether they are happy or not, should be very privileged. These features, which we take for granted, do not apply to everyone in the world. They are the exception, not the rule.

Secondly, if your main concern at the moment is happiness and personal fulfillment, you do not need basic things such as food, home, clothing, education, etc. To be included in happiness, you must be a privileged person who already has his or her basic human needs. People who live in poor poverty without, for example, political rights, do not wonder if they are happy. They think about how they want to feed their children and survive another day under an oppressive government regime. They don't have the luxury to pursue happiness. They pursue their fundamental human rights. This is not you.

There is a famous theory of self-actualization (which essentially means happiness) that was proposed by Abraham Maslow in 1943 as "A Theory of Human Motivation". It is most remarkable because of his hypothesis about the hierarchy of human needs to achieve personal fulfillment. These needs are structured in the form of a pyramid with basic human needs such as food, water, sex and homeostasis (control of body temperature and regulation of hormone activity) below and moral, creativity and lack of prejudice at the top.

Maslow stated that very few people are ever aware of self-actualization, and I usually agree with him. I don't think it's because we cannot achieve happiness and self-actualization. I think our inclusion of materialism, money, physical perfection, and our lack of self-discipline and spirituality, rather than our true needs, strays us. It is our need to nurture hurt and horror that disrupts our ability to function in a mentally healthy and effective manner.

This is not to deny your needs, desires and your dissatisfaction with the stress factors in your life. We have them all included and can be distracting and distracting. There are good reasons to be unhappy. Finding out that you have a terminal illness is devastating, especially if little can be done for you.

However, this is the end of the spectrum, and I will not address such concerns in this article because it is not its focus.It is the perspective of how fortunate it is to be so elusive, and therefore the reason we are so busy achieving it. Now you can be very happy and you don't even know it. There are certainly many reasons. Not sure what it is? I just mentioned ten for you and I'm willing to bet you can add a few more. Travel? Holiday? Physical fitness? Home enhancements for pure beauty? The list can continue.

The Dalai Lama has published numerous publications on how to achieve happiness through the basic things of Buddhism. If you are interested in pursuing an intangible and spiritual lifestyle while still satisfying your basic human needs, you may want to look at Buddhism. This religion emphasizes that happiness is based on the state of mind and the perspective of events and circumstances. The transformation of our attitudes and beliefs is the key to happiness.Your pursuit of happiness may be the result of a lack of spirituality in your life. Spiritually, I do not necessarily mean faith in God or becoming a member of organized religion.

Spirituality can be found in many wonderful forms, such as transcendentalism (focused on one's inner, mental nature), respect for nature, love for animals, artistic creativity and many other beliefs and practices that nourish your spirit and experience in the world. There are many forms of spirituality and less attention to our physical self and more to our recognition of the human mind can be an important part of achieving happiness.If I were to suggest a checklist of ways to decipher happiness here, it would look like this:

- Create your spirituality no matter what form you like
- Reduce the desire for wealth and material possessions
- Find meaningful and satisfying work
- Register as a volunteer and engage in community interactions to avoid focusing so much on you
- Watch full and fun hobby or fun
- Appreciate the many amazing features and privileges you have (see list above)
- Recognize the many gifts in your life, including your political rights, responsibilities and the freedom to strive for happiness
- See others
- Learn to forgive

TOP 5 RECOGNIZED TECHNIQUES FOR LEADING A TRULY HAPPY AND JOYFUL LIFE INDOORS AND OUTDOORS!

True happiness can be experienced by anyone who applies "habits of happiness" in his time. Some are just being born with a happy attitude. But the truth is; Most people have to learn to be happy by thinking and living in a certain way.People are often happy in life when everything goes well. But those who have learned to be happy are not always those who "have everything." The appearances do not affect their level of joy. They have discovered the secret that they can experience basic peace and well-being; which is the essence of true happiness.

Happy people live their lives differently. And when you acquire new skills, it pays to learn from professionals.Take a look at these five basic skills when you are ready to get some joy inside.

Top 5 recognized techniques for true happiness

1) Pay attention and thank you for the happy things in your life

Learn to notice everything well and positively in your life, no matter how small. What things do you see, feel, taste, hear, or feel that bring joy?

The intent activates a part of the brain, the reticular activation system (RAS), which is responsible for turning on our memory and allowing us to draw attention to something important. When you decide to look positive, your RAS ensures that this is what you see.

We tend to give birth to the unfortunate negative side of life. Make it a game to see how many good things you'll notice during the day. Take a moment and enjoy the positive things and make the habit of nourishing your happiness.

2) Do not believe everything you think

Don't believe everything you think. Our thoughts are not always correct.

For example, you can make a presentation and focus on a person with a frown on his face and think you are doing very well. Yet the fact is that you are doing well, but the rest of the group doesn't smile and nods.It is said that we average a second for thinking in our lessons, and the vast majority are the usual negative thoughts. This gale of automatic negative thoughts can stimulate parts of the brain that include depression and anxiety.

Learn not to believe in a negative idea that wants to bear your happiness, and instead focus on positive compliments. It is important to break the natural tendency to register negative thoughts, feelings and experiences deeper than positive ones.

3) Change a bad idea to a happy one

When dealing with negative, unhappy thoughts and feelings in a situation, you must learn to exchange them for equally true, positive and happy thoughts.

E.g. Have you ever had a deadline and do you think it was not possible to finish on time? Why not exchange a self-confident idea by searching in my mind for a positive idea like I can get things on time regularly and ask for help.

Learn to be more optimistic and see the glass half full. Pay more attention to the positive part of the truth in your situation and rely on these ideas. May your strength be the joy of the Lord.

4) Appreciate people in your life

People with good social relationships are usually happy. In times of stress, we need the support of friends and family. And the best way to keep relationships happy and healthy is through appreciation.

By showing others recognition of the support they provide, we reinforce this behavior; which in turn deepens our relationship with them. Engaging and communicating with others in times of stress has a calming effect and keeps us on the road to happiness.

5) Live with passion and sense

A sense of sense and passion for your daily activities will increase your happiness. Think about the activities in your life that interest you. What about the things that make you happy?

One person may feel an under-paid manager, but the other can do his job full of passion to make the building a great place for others.Learn to integrate purpose and passion into your daily life at work and home. Do everything with joy from the heart concerning the

Lord.The truth is, you don't have to let your life throw you in unfortunate waters. You can decide to learn new skills, live your life differently and increase your level of happiness.

TRUE FREEDOM - LIVING A LONG AND HEALTHY LIFE

It is not unusual that today we find people over the age of 90.As I get older, I wonder what I could or could do to live in a wonderfully mature age. What is even more important to me is that I wonder what I could or could not do to live well into old age.

Although I am not healthy, I do not find it useful to live for 70 years. This is the focus of this blog. I hope many young people will read and take note of this because now that you are young, the preparation for a good life must be done in recent years.After having been several times, I have noticed that many young people, especially men of our kind, tend to suffer from 'Super Hero' syndrome. They think they can do what they want and have no consequences.

So many young people are imprisoned by drinking alcohol and taking excessive medication, doing crazy things that raise their muscles, and doing poor maintenance by not eating well and not getting enough sleep.If the situation is getting worse when young people think they are insensitive to natural laws, and they show this by constantly performing the above activities. Damage is not necessarily committed by the act itself; the long-term effect is the lack of post-event maintenance.

As you often hear older people say, "Oh, it's just old football or hockey injury."

Would they have had such damage so many years later if they had taken the time to care for themselves? I do not think so!The youth seems to be doing crazy things to burn all the excess energy. But I don't worry if you go out and do things like extreme sports, go

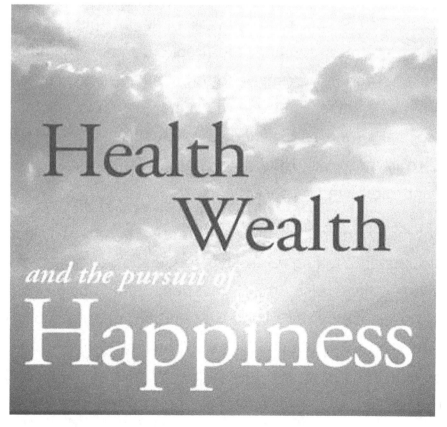

crazy in a skate park or make hot dogs your main diet, I strongly suggest you learn how to soften your choices by balancing your choices.

If you are watching your body, we recommend that you go to a session with a chiropractor or massage therapist to get your body back in line. With regular replenishment, you can continue these sports for much longer, and you don't have to have an "old football" injury later.The same is true for food, if you bite hot dogs and beer too much, your body will be affected by a lack of good food. Take a regular break and eat a balanced diet. If you smoke, give up, it just makes you old.

My specialty is to help people with belief systems that cause unnatural aging and even premature death.Unfortunately, most people do not understand that what they believe is true, not only may it not be true, but may even be harmful to their health and longevity.

We are not limited to the life that creates our faith!

We are free spirits who can make everything we want out of our lives. We just have to be willing to do the work to make changes and be ready to pay the price along the way. After all, it's usually just a fear of being released!If you think life is a big party and it is good to live on bad food, drugs, alcohol, and sleep deprivation, it will catch up with you and cause severe limitations as you get older.

It is important that if you recognize one of your beliefs that do not lead a healthy, happy and functional life, you will take the time to do something about it immediately. So many people can live in happier relationships, be more successful and live a much more exciting life if they take the time to do something about the dysfunctional beliefs we all have to deal with.How can you have a good relationship with another person if you believe that you will stay with you and say that you are not good enough?

How can you be successful in your career if you have a faith that tells you that the world wants to get you?

It is important if you want to live a long and healthy life that you are starting today to take better care of yourself. Take the time to get to know each other. Discover what drives you.

If you find something about yourself that makes you feel unhappy, do something about it. Follow the situation-related workshops, visit a counselor who can help or just make other decisions.

Remember what your life looks like is entirely based on how you think life is. If there is something in your life that is not good for you in a healthy way, change it.Every living person is here to live well now and in the long term. However, this requires some initiative and some effort to ensure that your decisions today offer a better future. If you are 80 years old, and yes, that day is coming, you will be glad you did it during the Boston Marathon!

Accept the mix (what Mom and Dad didn't know were taught)

Stress stamp

Monty's knowledge of psychology and personal attention is supported by his own life experiences and challenges that grow up in a dysfunctional environment as a child. Unable to accept the pain and discomfort of the outcome of his life, he embarked on his lifelong mission to understand his life and build a better life. As this process evolved, he began to write and teach practical ways to improve the quality of life for others. Monty's approach to addressing life issues is always practical and often out of the box from a mysterious than an academic point of view.

Here's how to live a healthy life by changing your habit

A healthy life is undoubtedly the greatest desire of us all. After all, without health, life radically changes its meaning. The best way to feel happy, energetic and healthy in the future is to live a happy, energetic and healthy life in the present. The benefits and joys produced are both immediate and long-term.

We are increasingly moving in a direction where people are finally realizing that being healthy is much more than just not being sick.

We cannot let life pass through us without living it with energy and stimuli that convey happiness to us. We need to make our lives more attractive and stimulating by simply taking a firm, active and participatory attitude towards them.

Many times we are unable to stop the journey of life. Despite this fact, life is also the fruit of our attitudes and behaviors. We are therefore the result of our experiences.

How to have a healthy life?

"What needs to be done to be healthy", "how to start a healthy life" or "how to have a healthy and happy life" are questions that people often ask themselves.

Debrucemo, first on the issue:

What does it mean to be healthy? According to the World Health Organization (WHO), health is "physical, mental and social well-being rather than the absence of disease ...". In other words, being healthy is not just the absence of disease, but essentially the physical and mental well-being of the individual. It is no coincidence that the WHO defines health in this way and gives the word a much broader meaning than mere antonyms of disease.

Although health seems to be naturally associated with the word medicine, it goes well beyond the sense that common sense often attributes to it, as it is usually associated only with medicinal drugs. But medicine is much more than that because it is primarily about disease prevention.

People's lifestyles, poor diet, stress, and other factors have contributed significantly to problems. Examples include diabetes and high blood pressure, diseases that are closely related to the habits of modern people.

Many of the problems that modern medicine helps to solve can be easily avoided if they are followed by some of the most important recommendations for practicing a healthy lifestyle.

Changing habits and behaviors is necessary and urgent. By this, we do not mean that we must adhere to the letter of all the rules of a healthy life as if it were a difficult, painful and even castrating plan for people. Life must be guided with intensity and joy, so we should never become mere prisoners of attitudes/behaviors that, although healthier, would be both painful and restrictive.

Life consists of possibilities. Take your consciousness, strike a balance between the pros and cons of your taste, towards a healthier life, and remember that ultimately you want to improve your quality of life.

We are talking about changing attitudes that stimulate us and lead us to happiness and thus improve our health. It is not always possible, it is true, but in the vast majority of cases, it is fully achievable.

For example, imagine a simple walk in the countryside or enjoy your favorite piece of fruit. These are two simple examples where you can enjoy life and improve your health at the same time.

Food, exercise

A healthy life is also in our hands. Let us not judge that we can eat too much sugar every day and that once we suffer from diabetes, it will simply be a matter of fate and bad luck. We cannot judge who is exposed to high doses of stress daily and we will not permanently pay a high price for it. We do not think we can smoke for years and not collect respiratory problems and impair our quality of life.

Our attitude reminds us of sooner or later about our health.

Of course, our attitude toward life is a decisive factor for a healthier life. Before the intervention, feel life positive and feel good about yourself.Keep in mind at least two important things. First, nutrition. A good diet can do much more for your health than you think. Nutrition and healthy life are inseparably linked concepts.

Second, physical exercise. The right way can greatly improve your health and well-being and thus contribute to a better quality of life.You see exercise as something positive and relaxing, not something difficult and "it should be". See which activity you like best and see the benefits it can offer.

Just change these two factors and discover a healthier life.

If you are going to delve deeper into these and other topics, we recommend reading our blog articles about nutrition and the benefits of exercise.

Quality of life

How many of us already feel discomfort caused by simple back pain. Or you may feel discomfort caused by recurrent infections, often caused by a weakening of our immune system.However, many of the examples we can point out are all aware that illnesses or discomforts drastically reduce our quality of life.

Today we live in an era where it is time to dictate the rules. Lack of time leads people to live in a constant race against this precious resource.We don't have time to eat well, we don't have time to exercise, we don't have time to talk to people, we don't have time to do many things that are considered essential in our lives. Unfortunately, this behavior presents several problems with serious consequences for our health and well-being.

In the presence of these problems, on the one hand, people are greatly affected by their health, on the other hand, their quality of life is greatly impaired.

In short, we would say that it is not possible to have a good quality of life without healthy habits.

Healthy life

Life expectancy a few decades ago was significantly lower.With the improvement of living conditions and progress in medicine is gradually increasing. Yet it is because we all want to live better and longer.

The current goal is not just to live longer. It is to have lasting health, that is, to lead an active, healthy, happy and purposeful life. However, living longer is not synonymous with a better life. The increase in life expectancy often comes at the expense of more or less sophisticated treatments that, despite their effectiveness, significantly harm people's quality of life. We should not just want to live more, but live better.Life is also in our hands. We are inevitably convinced that we must focus our attention on maintaining a healthy state, and our attitudes today will have a profound impact on our future health.

If you want to live healthier and longer, you need to start taking action in this direction, ie measures that are firm, healthy and contribute to your current health.

Benefits of a healthy life.

The benefits of a healthy life are innumerable. So it will not be necessary to describe them with the extractor, because we all know what is nice to feel healthy or, on the contrary, what is painful to feel bad.But the benefits of a healthy life are not over. Health care costs are becoming increasingly difficult for people, either directly or indirectly through taxes levied on the public health system.

Some studies clearly show that for every dollar invested in prevention, we can achieve a significant return on savings through medical treatment procedures.In other words, investment priority should be directed toward disease prevention. On the other hand, the social and economic costs of illness, such as absence from work, are very significant with rising social protection costs.

HEALTH AND WELLNESS

It is undeniable that today there is a great interest in healing health, where the drug has evolved enormously in recent years. As we have seen, these advances in medicine have undoubtedly brought people a longer life span and a better quality of life.

If there is no health, our whole life is shorter and we cannot live and taste it in its fullness.We must, therefore, think about our future, because our quality of life also reflects the way we live today.

Therefore, a new paradigm must emerge in which the promotion of health and a stronger approach of people to the prevention of diseases with huge health benefits that improve their quality of life and well-being. In short, each of us is supposed to develop a healthier lifestyle where health is paramount.For all these reasons, we inevitably believe that the commitment to disease prevention, health promotion, and well-being is paramount.

For a healthy life

When you are ready to focus on weight loss and

fitness, we will discuss three aspects of healthy living that are courage, change, and choice.

An easy way to remember 3 c of a healthy life is with this simple sentence: to develop a healthy life you need to have the courage to change the choices you encounter. Sounds like something you're interested in? Let's dive into each of these topics to see what they mean, so you can be as successful with this often difficult business.

The 3 Cs in a healthy life

The courage to develop a healthy life

One of the first most important basic needs for developing a healthy life is courage. Courage is of the utmost importance because you face several problems that will make you feel uncomfortable. You will intentionally force yourself to address problems that you have probably avoided in the past, and that is why you have achieved the amount of weight that you have today.

For example, you must have the courage to get off the couch, put on some tennis shoes, and go outside to walk or run for an hour 3-5 days a week. You must have the courage to make healthy food for lunch or dinner in your kitchen. It takes a lot of courage to manage effective weight loss daily.

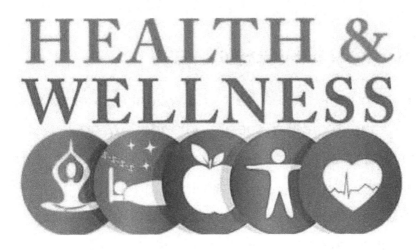

Change to a healthy life

Once you have decided that you dare to do this weight loss process fairly, the next point in the company is to make changes in your life. Weight gain is generally the result of absorbing far too many calories than your body needs regularly and does not consistently get enough exercise. These are the specific areas that need to be addressed and turned into moments that are beneficial to your health.

You must be willing to change some aspects of your life if you want to have a chance to lose weight successfully. Switch from soft drinks to water. Switch from huge fast-food meals to home-made meals with the right portions. Switch from potato snacks to almonds with raisins. These are the changes that you need to have courage.

Possibilities of healthy life

Once you dare to deal with the weight loss process and are willing to make specific changes to how you live your life, the last step is to address the many options you face every day. This can be the hardest part of all this effort because there are a lot of options that you need to do every day.

Think of everything that has happened today since you woke up this morning. There were probably 5 to 10 choices in terms of diet and exercise that you had to take because you got out of bed. Here are some likely choices you have described:

- Do I have to get up early to apply?
- What should I eat?
- Do I have to eat a snack while watching TV?
- What's my lunch?
- Do I have to get anything out of the machine during the break?
- Stop from work home and pick up a portion of fast food or pizza?

- Snacks on a chip bag while driving to work?

Each of these options affects your weight loss efforts. The effect will be positive if you make guided and conscientious decisions. The effect may be negative if you do not maintain self-control and strong willpower.It's all on your shoulders to make the right choices that will benefit your health and then help you lose weight. This process takes time, so stick to 3 Cs of healthy life to reach your goal.

Living a healthy life can even lead to a longer life

No matter how hectic your daily schedule may be, always keep in mind that having the right amount of rest is very important to give your body energy the next day. This way you can recover your energy and be ready for the next day. Health experts now believe that regular exercise along with your other activities and proper bleaching can lead to a longer life. You can add more years to your life simply by practicing your health style.

One of the best things that can help improve your mental and physical condition is laughter. It is said that laughter is the best medicine. People are automatically attracted to someone who has a good sense of humor.

Always remember that you can also create a sense of humor and a positive outlook by surrounding yourself with happy people.

On the other hand, you have to realize that stress is not good for your health. The only thing that causes stress is disturbing. You should know that stress can lead to serious health problems such as severe headache, asthma, high blood pressure, stomach problems, heart condition and the like.

Regular exercise will always be part of a healthy life. People must exercise a lot, especially for those who do not maintain a balanced diet. By physical fitness you look good and feel good, giving you confidence.A healthy exercise program will help slow the aging process. Therefore, it is recommended to do something physical every day. If you don't use your collections, you'll only get a curved and worn outlook, because they naturally tighten when they are rarely used. When we think about old age, we often see a bent look.

If you want to maintain a healthy body and mind, it is important to eat the right food, have a good rest and relax. These habits must work hand in hand if you want to live a healthy life all the time, which can lead to a longer, happier and above all a completed life.

4 tips for a healthy life

Living a healthy life is the primary goal of many. With all the excitement and stress in your home, work, and school environment, you can be one of many people wondering how they can lead a healthy life.

Living a healthy life has many different factors. It's not just about physical well-being, because that's just one aspect of your multifaceted life. You are here not only to exist but also to change. To do this, you must be healthy and lead a healthy life.

Here are four different steps you can take to lead a healthy life:

1. Your emotional health is as important as your physical health

The basic question you can ask is: how can I express my feelings? Some so many people keep the emotions suspended inside until they can no longer hold them, which in turn leads to emotional and physical disturbances. The art is to express yourself. Do not be afraid to express your anger or strong feelings because there are positive ways to do this. You can write it if you can't say it. You can also correct the person who did the wrong thing by talking to him about the problem. Remember, when it comes to emotional health, it pays to express what you feel.

2. A healthy life begins from within

Learn to love yourself. You certainly have strengths and weaknesses; talent and weakness. You must learn to accept these attributes because they will be part of you throughout your life. On the one hand, you must first acknowledge your weaknesses to overcome them. On the other hand, use your strengths to further sharpen them. Socrates said, "Know yourself." Only by knowing yourself will you love who you are and what you are.

3. A healthy life requires a healthy diet and an active lifestyle

Fast food is not healthy food. With the hustle and bustle of urban life, people often go to fast food chains to eat meals. But don't even bite this habit. Cook food at home and take it to work or school. Eat less meat and more vegetables; fewer carbohydrates and more fiber. Moreover, a healthy diet is not enough. It must be combined with training. Plan the training plan that works best for you. One of the most popular and easy to do exercises is fast walking, jogging, the-bo and even dancing. So get up and burn some calories!

4. Be grateful for the little things life gives

There is nothing healthier than a grateful heart. Learn to appreciate small blessings such as walking through the park or being with your loved ones for dinner. These are small things that make life more meaningful. The more you focus on positive things, the more you enjoy life. It is also easier to overcome obstacles when you think positively.

Checklist items to confirm yourself

Whether everything you want to do is daunting and stressful.I think we have reached the saturation point. We live in a busy world where everything goes fast. In our gallop with many tasks, we are exhausted. It's time to launch. We must stop constant movement and strive to be all for all. We must stop paying attention to everything and anyone who needs it.

Wait a while. Breathe. Stop and breathe right now. Place your hand on your stomach and breathe deeply. Breathe deep enough to raise your hand. Here's how to breathe. But most of the time we don't breathe that way. Some of us never breathe this way. If you are under stress, your breathing will be lower. There is not enough oxygen in the brain and organs and you are tired or ill. Do you want to live your life like this?

It is time for us to create space in our lives for what is important. We have to do so much and we want so much, not everything will inevitably happen. Let's stop going crazy and focus on what's important.

Taking care of your health is the most important step towards a happy life. It does not matter how much money you have, because without good health you cannot enjoy and care for the people and things that are most important to you.

We intend to lead a happy and healthy life. The visualization takes a few seconds. You have to move and breathe easily. You must feed yourself with healthy food and healthy activities. You have to feel calm and healthy every day. And wherever you are in the continuum, you can start a happier and healthier life today. Strengthen yourself. Take control. Decide that you are important and from now on you will take care of yourself and your health. Your life and the lives you touch every day benefit from your good health.

We have been in a "rush" state for so long that it is difficult for many people to figure out how to slow down. A good way to start is to find out how you spend your days. Look honestly at how you spend every minute every day. We have often developed habits that no longer make sense. Have a look at your activities and ask yourself, does this activity have more benefits for me? Does anyone else use it? If you are honest with yourself, you will find that many of these things are unnecessary or can be done by anyone else. Removing only a few of these unnecessary activities can create additional space for your day. The purpose is not to immediately fill these moments with more work. The goal is to create space for your health. Once you have lost your time, you can create a life of good health and joy with the following actions.

Sleep is one of the keys to health. It can be preferred. Turn off the TV. Leave the job. It can wait. If it is not enough to sleep, it can influence our decision-making, our mood, our creative thinking and let us weigh even more. Studies have shown that lack of sleep reduces the regulation of hormones that control our appetite. Think about the moments when you felt unusually hungry and carbohydrate after a night's sleep. Set a reasonable bedtime and stick to it. Your reward is fresh thinking, fresher skin, and more energy.

Take time to drink plenty of water. This promotion is so simple but so important. Stay hydrated to wash away toxins, have healthier skin and support your metabolism. We are often wrong with a hunger for hunger, so if you drink enough water, you can control the amount you eat.

Take a good multivitamin. Along with water and the right amount of sleep, you will be amazed at changing energy levels.Whatever you do every hour, get up for a while, stretch and move. We didn't have long to sit at desks and computers or anywhere else. Stretching, movement, mind.

Show gratitude every day. Acknowledgment is a de-stressor that makes you feel good. Negative thoughts cause stress. It is difficult to have negative thoughts and gratitude thoughts in our minds.

Take time for friends. Healthy relationships help us stay healthy. This does not mean that you must accept each invitation. Give yourself time to think about your invitation response. Is this something you want to do? Would you regret giving up your sleep or time with your family or wife? Sometimes parties are not where we want to be. We are overwhelmed by food and drink and the next day we punish other calories we have consumed and the fatigue we feel.

How you spend minutes daily contributes to how you spend your life. The way you live your life and the decisions you make determine how healthy and strong you want to be. Do you make decisions that will strengthen or weaken you? If you make decisions that make you happy and healthy, it's great and I say, keep it! If not, you can choose another method. Happy, healthy way.

GOLDEN RULES FOR A HEALTHY LIFE

If we want to have a healthy body, it is necessary to give everything it needs. The way we live and the way we think about ourselves is also an important aspect of our well-being. The golden rules of healthy living are a guide for a good life.

- Be gentle. (Don't eat too much.)
- Don't miss breakfast.
- Never go out with an empty stomach.
- Eat different kinds of quality food.
- Always compensate for lost fluid.
- Respect the rest of the night.
- You should be active.
- Expose today and fresh air.
- Develop a spirit of optimism and goodwill.

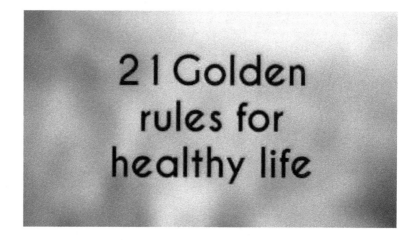

Why is each of these rules important?

Moderation means that we behave in a way that does not expose our bodies to extreme challenges, especially for a long time. For example, we must try to avoid many of the harmful substances we eat in our daily lives, such as (coffee, alcohol, tobacco, preservatives, flavor enhancers). If you are depressed, it is undoubtedly useful to drink a glass of wine or a good piece of chocolate after a good meal, but nothing more.

People who skip breakfast have more weight problems because they interfere with the natural rhythm of their metabolism.When we are hungry, we are tempted to eat something. If we continue, we go home even more and go to everything that happens to us uncontrollably. It is therefore good to always have fresh fruits and vegetables at home.

The quality of the food and drink we consume determines the quality of our health. For example, fibers cleanse the body of harmful substances; certain foods stimulate metabolism; Carbohydrates are the first energy source for muscles and proteins as their most important structural material is the most valuable energy source. As we age, our bodies lose calcium, bones become weak, and it is very important to take enough calcium when we are young.

Fluid balance is one of the main causes of some diseases. Our bodies can lose approximately every day. 10 glasses of liquid, even if we do nothing. We must compensate for this loss and the best way to do this is to consume freshwater.The only time our body is restored is when we sleep. We need to have enough sleep hours to benefit. Sleep well and live long.

Regular exercise reduces the risk of serious illness. The study claims that four hours of training a day. Week reduces breast cancer incidence by 66.6%. Running is good for the heart and lungs and also improves brain function by increasing oxygen supply.

Sunlight is the source of every life. It helps our vital organs to be strong and function properly. With fresh air, we inhale the energy and oxygen of nature that is needed to burn calories, which optimizes our body functions.Most of us want to live the same way and eat the same food as before and use a pill that magically solves their problems. But the solution is in us. If our mind is focused on good things, we do good things. By identifying with a successful team, we can develop a competitive spirit. The quality of our lives seems to be better when there is more harmony in our family and we have friends. The best way to get rid of stress is to live in a simple and relaxed way.

Why is it important to use this set of golden rules?

Medicines help the body overcome health problems, but medications cannot cure the causes. The cause of the disease is not the absence of drugs, but a violation of the rules of a healthy life. If we want to enjoy a healthy life, we just have to fight through the golden rules of a healthy life that we value most.

Here you can read how you can have a successful relationship to help you lead a healthy life.Build healthy relationships with your beloved friends and those; Maybe with their parents, young children, adult children, husband, former spouses, cousins, golf friend, etc.?

The Metaphysical Principles of the Miracle Course help us see the light of a healthy life through healthy and sacred relationships.Believe it or not, there is clinical evidence that recommends that our relationships can truly contribute to a healthy life and minimize disease and illness. Therefore, the fundamental goal is that our relationship is healthy to achieve a healthy life.A miracle course says, "This is the time of faith. You have set this goal for you."

There have been studies to recommend that married people tend to live longer.

A healthy life

Professionals believe that building healthy relationships, especially in marriage, provides a nurturing environment for people, allowing them to fight against diseases better.

Supporting a loving spouse can make a difference in the world, especially when it comes to a serious illness.Building healthy relationships can help reduce anxiety and stress. Excitement is believed to be a major cause of illness.

How you can have a successful relationship can be a nice goal by implementing healthy relationship tips that seem to end up for you and further improve your relationships with other people.A miracle course further says: "Don't you think that the very purpose of joy is to arrange the means for achieving it?

Healthy conditions tips

This is especially the case with family members - where we can minimize the tension that can ease our strength, making it difficult for us to ward off infections.It is not enough to know that building healthy relationships can make us much healthier. It is also very important to know exactly how we can ensure that we have a healthy relationship.

Psychologists claim that interaction is the most important active ingredient in a healthy relationship.

Try to understand your desires and goals before you interact with your relationships. To put it simply, you must understand exactly what you want before you articulate it to another person.

Try to keep an open mind and listen carefully to what the other person is trying to discuss.

Be judgmental

If you are angry with someone's habits, try not to judge or criticize: "You are always late." Instead, say something to the result: "If you're gone and I don't hear from you, I worry."

In this way, you tell the other how you feel through his

/ her behavior. It is also important that you admit your mistakes and apologize for that.Such a basic act shows that you are concerned about the feelings of the other.Building healthy relationships also depends on limiting yourself and respecting the limits of other people. You should never tolerate abuse in a relationship, physically or emotionally.

Reduce stress and anxiety

To achieve a healthy life, it is important to make our relationship healthy.Remember that building healthy relationships can help reduce stress and anxiety, leading to stress that is not good for a healthy life.

It is not enough to understand that building healthy relationships can make us healthier, but it is also very important to know exactly how we can guarantee successful relationships.

BUILDING A HAPPY LIFE: 10 MOST IMPORTANT INGREDIENTS

If you ask most people what their biggest goals in life are, it sounds like this: Living a happy and productive life where I feel I want to change the lives of others. Many of us are produced in our lives and we make a difference in the lives of others, but it seems that the most important component - happiness - is missing. The following tips help create more happiness in your life:

1) Find something passionate about it. What drives you? What motivates you? What gives you meaning and purpose in life? If you want happiness in life, you must be able to answer these questions. Insignificant; purposes; something that is passionate about it - life can be outdated and boring. Outdated white bread is unlikely to make most people happy.

2) Simplify your life. Remove your house and your life. If possible, take a week off work and go through each room in the house. Cans or trash bags marked, discarded and distributed. Remove things you no longer use or have not used in the last 12 months. If you have projects that you have not completed, make

sure you drop or complete those projects even if you are out of work. If you cannot take time off from work, take time each night or weekend and walk through each room.

3) Set goals you want to achieve. Having a goal and achieving it brings a sense of satisfaction. A sense of satisfaction or pride in a well-executed task often implies some happiness in life. If we live our lives without goals, we are often lost and life begins to feel bad. We get stuck and start to feel miserable and helpless. Having a goal, set or goal development helps us stay on the road in life.

4) Start some traditions in your life. What pleased you as a child? Can you now incorporate this into your life? When I was little I loved the vacation. My mother had a lot of cookie cutters that we would draw for each holiday season. We make Halloween cookies, Thanksgiving cookies, Christmas cookies, Valentine cookies, you get it. It was a nice tradition. Now I'm doing it with my daughter. It's a sticky time and a chance to be happy when baking and decorating cookies. You don't have to wait and have children or a family to build traditions. With your friends, you can plan an annual trip for walks, sightseeing or shopping.

It's something you do every year where you can relax and have fun in your life.

5) In addition to establishing traditions, it is important to establish contact with others. If you just work and go home and watch TV, life gets bored pretty quickly. If you are an introvert and a new member of the area where you live, look for a nonprofit where you can volunteer. If you're more social, browse your local weekly newspaper for the clubs that meet. I live in the suburbs of a larger city. There is every kind of club that people can join. When I lived in a smaller area, there were still ways to become a member - join a fitness group or gym, go to a local leisure center for an art course - there are plenty of places to connect with people. You just have to look.

6) Compare with your neighbor (or anyone else). Accept your uniqueness and celebrate your individuality. There are certain things in your life that you can never change, so try to stop. By the way, you never know what's going on in the house/life of your neighbor or friend. For example, you might be jealous of how lean and fit your friend is, and yet you don't know that she has been fighting bulimia and bad faith for years. Whether the best house in your area is filled

with anger and hatred tied together in a nasty divorce.

7) Be responsible for yourself. Stop waiting for the perfect companion, the perfect job, the perfect set of friends who can fill your life with meaning. No one else can make you "whole" or fill your life with "meaning". Only you can do it. If you want a happy life, find out what happiness means to you and take steps to build it in your life.

8) Ensure sufficient rest. Some people find it difficult to be happy when they walk all day with a lack of sleep. Good sleep is important to our overall health. We must make good decisions and spend our day effectively.

9) Eat well. In addition to good rest, it is important to eat a healthy diet. Too much sugar and caffeine can cause not only physical but also emotional.

10) Choose whether you want to be happy. If you do not choose, you will not be happy in life. Happiness doesn't come to you continuously. It requires you to make conscientious decisions in your life. Just allowing life doesn't lead to the maximum amount of happiness you can have.

Looking for the deep secrets of a happy life? Test yourself

If you are looking for the true meaning of happiness in life, your search is over because you will discover the deep secret of a happy life.

Below are six important questions that you should know if you are interested in discovering the deep secrets of a happy life. These questions and the supply analysis will provide you with the right answer.

1. Why should I be happy to be happy:

- It is the cornerstone of a happy life
- You become selfish
- This is not important to you

The real answer is here A. Because you can't be happy in any way unless you're really in love. True happiness comes from knowing that you love yourself and that when you can spread the same love to others. And it supports it saying that "if you don't love yourself, why would anyone go for it?" Happiness and living a happy life are about loving oneself and ultimately others forming the basis for a happy life.

2. Influence your people to be happy:

- It has nothing to do with happiness
- You will be happy and create networks of happy friends
- Allows you to navigate a separate path

The answer is B. It has been said that "you can have more friends in two weeks if you are interested than in two years if you want to be interested in you" and that brings you happiness. The famous author David Niven Ph.D. notes this in his book 100 Simple Mysteries of Happy People and states that he is noble: "Friendship is one of the most important joys of life." usually the joy of life comes from memories of the moment shared with those we love in our hearts. When you do this, you will eventually find a group of people who can maintain a relationship that allows you to be extremely yourself.

3. Why should I learn to risk being happy:

- Happiness, which is an internal joy, is accompanied by risk-taking
- (b) You don't have to risk being happy
- (c) Happiness is not risk-taking

The answer is A. The joy and satisfaction that life brings can easily be ascribed to the leap of faith that is needed to achieve your goals. Therefore, it is said that the happiest people on Earth are those who are not afraid to take risks. Risking is associated with the challenge of the status quo, doing things you've ever dreamed of in the corner of your house that makes you happy, things like diving in the sky; embark on a trip you've always dreamed of; talk to your beloved high school; apply for an advanced job you were always afraid of; do something wrong and you are certainly happy about life.

4. Ensure flexible benchmarking for a happy life:

- Having a plan is not enough
- Having a plan is not a guarantee of happiness
- Having a plan that is S.M.A.R.T and flexible is good luck

The correct answer is C. It has already been stated without numbers that "If you do not intend to fail". To be happy, you have to plan it, it just doesn't happen by accident. How satisfied are you with the specific talents you want on your S.M.A.R.T. Plans ensure long-term happiness. Therefore, to a happy life, step by step according to your plan and enjoy the moment they come.

5. I am happy in life when I have great wealth

(a) The great fortune you are unhappy with

(b) Become content and no wealth gives you luck

(c) Wanting more leads to greed

The real option is B. Here's the reason. Content or persistent content is the best way to be happy. Happy people think less about what they don't have, but stay happy and happy with what they already have. Because we are in a world of materiality where the great possession of material things and luxurious lifestyles seems to symbolize happiness, but often not, and this famous proverb has taken them all together, the "rich also cry" Life is often associated with the sport but easy to forget becomes life. It will surprise without surprise, and it also gives a surprise party! So be satisfied; term high; follow your dreams, but BE CONTENT!

6. How can I be happy?

- Happiness is a choice
- No one can make you happy
- Life itself can make you happy

The correct answer is A. A company called "TOTAL" has a stamp in one of its TV newsletters with the text "totally free choice", it can turn into reading, the happiness of choice. If you want to live a happy life, you decide to always be happy and decide every day to strengthen your belief system and start seeing that you live by what you have done. Choosing joy is more because it is related to the constant selection of these conscious decisions that will bring you happiness. As soon as it fits into your consciousness, you will come to life to make decisions that will make you no longer happy and because happiness is a choice and will gradually learn about these great decisions. happy life.

Live the truth about a happy life

Unfortunately, the world is full of unhappy people who want to live a happy life. Fortunately, most of these people can be happier if they lose existing misconceptions about happiness. It is easy for people to blame their happiness or lack of life aspects and not to take control of it. Take the time to read the following information to get better control and lose these misconceptions.

One of the biggest things that make people unhappy is money. Many people assume that you need money to be happy. However, if you look at it, you will find that money does not satisfy us. Rich people do not necessarily lead a happy life, and poor people are not always unhappy. When you open your eyes to the people around you, you will see it for yourself.

As long as they take care of your basic life needs, money is not important. Money can even make us unhappy, especially if we lose our lives by getting rich. We will often spend too much time working and neglecting the people around us. Many people find happiness because they know their family is happy and healthy with a full belly, clean clothes on their backs and a roof over their heads. Love, friendship and laughter are more important than anything that can be bought.

Unfortunately, another misconception that many think is that happiness makes us happy. Living a happy life is not about happiness. It's just to open up and make us happy, followed by happiness. Everyone has the opportunity to be happy, but they have to let themselves feel.

The last misconception is that people need others to be happy. But the truth is that you are responsible for your happiness and no one else can make you happy. Yes, having special people in life can contribute to happiness, but that's not the most important factor.

It is extremely difficult to be happy and to enjoy a happy life if these misconceptions appear in your head. You don't need money, you don't need other people, and you don't need happiness to make yourself happy. You are responsible for your destiny and your happiness, so control and live a happy life.

How to live a happy life

You will be happy, but this is not easy. You must learn to pursue happiness if you want to find it in life.

What is luck?

Happiness is safety, peace, love, glory, vision, wisdom, satisfaction and achievement.How can you achieve this goal? How can your life be characterized by perfect harmony?

You live in a crazy world ruled by terror and violence, where justice is just a game. On the other hand, you have inherited absurdity in most of your brain. To find happiness, you must find balance. You must also protect yourself against the dangerous world.

You cannot find happiness in life without sensitivity and sensitivity. You will inevitably encounter many obstacles during your journey.Without understanding how other people think and feel, you will make many mistakes in judging their behavior. You need special knowledge.If you just pursue happiness in life without having a plan, you will probably fail. It is hard to find happiness in life, even if you are seriously trying to achieve that goal. Now imagine how impossible it is to find real happiness in life without any organization.

You must work out a wise plan if you want to live a happy life.However, how can you work out a perfect life plan if you are so ignorant? This is impossible. Your plan will have many unreal parts based on assumptions that are far from the truth.How can you predict the future? How can you know in advance which way will help you find the treasure you are looking for?

There is a magical solution to all these problems and many other problems not mentioned here. The scientific method of dream interpretation, discovered by Carl Jung and simplified by me, helps you to immediately understand the word of God in dreams. All dreams are produced by the divine unconscious mind. Once you have mastered the dream language, you can understand God's guidance.

The divine unconscious mind that produces your dreams is the mind of God. God lives and sends you important messages in dreams to help you find healthy mental health, peace, love, and happiness. You just have to obey the unconscious guide to triumph in all aspects of life.

The unconscious mind shows you two fateful destinations in your dreams: the good destination and the bad destination that awaits you, depending on your actions. You also understand what you need to do to follow your positive destiny.

The unconscious mind is very generous and gives you a lot of explanation on all questions and answers all your questions in dreams. You also have information about the psychological state of others. You can predict the future and prepare the desired future results. You have unlimited benefits in coming into contact with divine wisdom.

You will learn how to strive for happiness by preparing appropriate living conditions for your success. This preparation involves transforming your personality and developing your sensitivity and sensitivity through dream therapy. You'll also learn how you can help your people find happiness through your actions.

THE KEY TO A HAPPY LIFE IS HOW YOU VIEW IT

What is happiness? Happiness is when we feel emotionally good. What also makes us feel good is the definition of satisfaction.People define happiness under different conditions to describe what is good for them. It can be excitement, fulfillment, passion, enthusiasm, love or freedom. For others, it can be a sense of satisfaction, hope or feel comfortable.

It can be your happiness or shared happiness with family members, friends or even strangers.Yet happiness is a state of mind. As Abraham Lincoln once said, "Most people are probably as happy as they are aware of." What does that mean?

For me, it is the satisfaction of what we have, where you live, alone or with someone else who is a partner in life or perhaps a family member or friend. We can make decisions and make it a reality so that she can live a happy life. Like what Mr. Lincoln hinted, if we were happy, we were in a state of happiness.Being happy in the present, just living, inspired by the goodness of everyone and counting all the blessings in life, is happiness.

But whether we define happiness or how we look at it, it feels good!

Let me quote another famous rule, this time from Aristotle. He once said, "Happiness depends on us." Therefore, happiness does not depend on other people or on having someone in your life with you or having all material possessions, such as expensive clothes, jewelry, high-tech aids, cars, etc.

We have to decide what makes us feel happy.

There are a few tricks for me. First, look for a quiet place where you can be alone. Some may argue what if there is no quiet place? I suggest every area where you can close the door or pull the curtain or imaginary curtain. Noisy around you? The most important thing you need to do now breathes deeply, close your eyes, and drown the sound by thinking of nothing but goodness and all your blessings throughout your life. Try to fill your mind with things that will please you, such as butterflies, wildflowers, barefoot running on the beach, watching the sunset, listening to your favorite radio program or anything that makes you smile.This thinking is very important in eliminating any unpleasant or painful feelings we have in the past or present.

Besides, forget about past mistakes, forgive people who have done the wrong thing, and forgive yourself. Leave the fallen away. Only then can we attain a state of happiness.I decide to be in a state of happiness, whatever comes my way. I could cry if I am sad or if I am injured. But I will stand up bravely, wipe the tears from my face and fill my mind with all the beautiful things that make me happy.

Important things in life

The time we live in today is very difficult and stressful. People easily get lost in their thoughts about priorities and what's important. It is very easy to fall into the trap of competing with your friend, neighbor or relative who has more money, a better car, home, nicer clothes or something else instead of taking care of your happiness and help others, you need to feel good and live a better life. This leads you to pursue money and forget to pay attention to people, spend time with your family, call your parents, and visit them and friends you don't have time for.

The recipe could be to stay focused. People should not neglect any part of their lives, but try to find balance and remind themselves from time to time of what has been left out, or perhaps for which too much has been taken, and therefore have bad consequences.

If you are a parent, you must already know how difficult that part is. However, in the interest of your children, you must be aware that you cannot be perfect because there is no such thing. What you can do is to love your children. Trying to give them a normal life, as I say to my children, with a lot of sleep, lots of fun and play, eating regularly and even sweets is cool, but only if they have eaten enough vegetables, fruit and everything they need to grow up to be strong and healthy adults. Too many toys and too many wishes do not always come out best for children, so you have to be in balance there too. What sport can do for children is great. It not only helps to develop their small bodies correctly, but also to teach them how to win, lose, make friends, and be persistent. All these things are things that help a child to be normal, mentally strong and ready for situations that one day's life entails.

Your job is another part of your life that can bring you joy or hell. Connecting with different people is only complicated if you take everything personally if you play situations and conversations in your head over and over again. You have to relax and free your mind.

If someone wants to fight, let them fight themselves. Do your job well, be honest and don't care for other unhappy and unstable people. They must try to free their mind, but that is not your problem.

Happiness is in us, but if we are out of the way and not aware of it, and if we always want something else to be happy, we are lost. Being happy is thinking more than anything. So take the time to see what you have, who you have and make your happy life around it. Being positive means that other people feel attracted to you so that you are surrounded by friends and that you are never alone and desperate and off the road again. People in your life will help you recover if you get lost; forget your priorities and what's important.

Here's your health: fitness is the key to a happy life

Fitness is the key to a happy life. I know many of you are rolling your eyes at this statement, but it's true. Leading an unhealthy lifestyle will lead to misery and unhappiness. This article will hopefully inspire you to start your fitness program so you can lose weight, build muscle and start a healthy lifestyle.

There is nothing but the thrill of excitement when the impossible is overcome. As home fitness videos get more intense, we may think we can't do these workouts. I remember that when I started the P90X and Insanity workouts, I would stop every so often to catch my breath because I was out of shape. Performing this kind of training reminded me of the days when I played football for the Highland Rams. During football season, our weight training would be Monday, Tuesday, Thursday and Friday. It was Wednesday that everyone was scared because we knew it was a sweat day. We would run for an hour through the stadium steps or do cardio and plyometric workouts, but I was in the best shape of my life in high school.

The secret to success with any form of training is that you must first overcome self-doubt. This is the most important key to having the body that you want. Secondly, if you go through the training, it's fine to stop and breathe and then get back into action. Don't beat yourself up if you have to stop often during training. Because over time you become stronger and faster and you can complete the training without stopping.

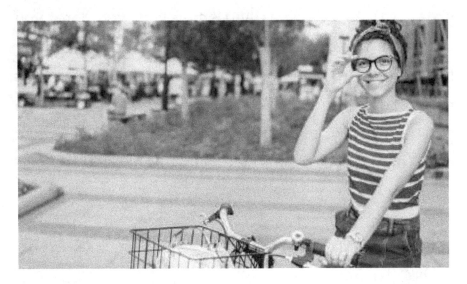

Third, set a goal for yourself and reward yourself with a treat when that goal is complete. These training sessions today are not a walk in the park. Fourth, make sure you eat a good, healthy meal because your body must be given the right nutrition to keep you working throughout the day.

If your workout allows fruit consumption, I would advise you to make a fruit smoothie so that you can get the right carbohydrates to burn your muscles. With this smoothie, I always make mine a combination of bananas, strawberries, apple, oranges, and blueberries with a slight addition of fresh leaf spinach (due to the large amounts of iron that the spinach contains). Throw them in a blender with a cup full of water and ice (add some liquid or stevia powder to sweeten the smoothie if desired). Mix them all and enjoy it. If you dare, you can make a vegetarian smoothie, but I prefer to drink high-potassium and low-sodium V8. Some workouts require that you go six days a week, while others go every other day, but regardless of the period, you must make an effort to reach the body you want.

ASTROLOGY TO BE HAPPY - HOW TO LIVE A HAPPY LIFE WITH ASTROLOGY

The origins of astrology date back to around 2900 BC People consider it a devout belief in certain forces that affect our lives. Some people think that astrology is a science. It can be defined as the art and science in the study of human-earth relationships. The positions, aspects, and movement of the sun, moon and eight planets are also leading for astrology.All the above movements have a major impact on human life.

Most people believe that astrology can predict the future. However, it is necessary to view this science as an incredible tool that can help you find the essence of life. The study of astrology and your birth chart by experts lets you learn the skills, qualities, and talents that you have brought into this world from past lives. This further helps you to share these qualities and contribute your skills to the well-being of this world. The planets have different qualities of energy and they influence a person's life in different ways.Astrology helps you lead a happy and peaceful life. Experts in this field believe that the character under which each person was born was assigned for a reason.

The cause becomes visible as you get older and his / her talents and qualities contribute to this world. Astrology is a path that leads us to goals to enrich our lives. These measures are effective in creating a better and happier life for ourselves.

Astrology directs us to people who are compatible with us and allows us to choose friends who can be long-term companies. Astrology compatibility analysis leads us to true love for our lives. This is the best way to live a happy marriage.

One of the greatest influences of astrology in our lives is the birth certificate. The symbols of development, transit, and progression in the birth chart allow us to visualize the activities and circumstances that await us in the near future. One can effectively analyze the period in which certain problems are most likely to occur in our lives. For example, the March Pluto rule is a crystal clear indication of the onset of anger and assertion problems in the near future.

The birth chart in astrology can predict the child's potential to perform certain activities in his or her life.

The negative and positive characteristics of a child can also be explored by this science.

This will help you explore the possibilities in your child's life. You can also choose an educational pattern or career for your child using predictions from your child's birth card.

There is a great significance of heavenly bodies and planets in our lives. Astrology believes that these elements govern different activities in a person's life and even tend to transform certain things that happen in someone's life. The sun is responsible for our trust and contributes to our success. A weak sun is an indication of a blurred and boring existence. The moon controls our emotions and is usually happy and satisfied in life. Mars facilitates us to move forward and achieve our goals. Mercury influences intelligence, communication and our potential to live a happy life. Jupiter is our teacher and Venus keeps us in a harmonized position. Saturn is a difficult planet and lets us perform our duties routinely. It is usually understood as the mourning and detachment planet.

Astrology has a huge impact on our lives. It is important to understand science instead of being afraid of it. If you understand the meaning of astrology in life, you can live a happy and prosperous life.

Appreciation and gratitude - the keys to a happy life?

Gratitude is fashionable. Not that there was ever a time when gratitude was not part of your life (hopefully), but at that time, when you open a book, blog or bag that relates to spirituality or personal growth, you'll probably find someone referring to how good to give gratitude and how it will attract all the possible benefits in your life. Appreciation is less fashionable, but in my opinion, it is just as important. So what are they, what are the differences and why are they so important for a happy life?

Gratitude and appreciation are essentially two sides of the same coin. And that coin is love. First, let's look at gratitude.

Gratitude is about giving - giving love in the form of thanks. When you give gratitude, you are grateful for something that has happened or that has come into your life and you express it. You can do it by word or in writing or through your promotions. Of course, it is one thing to thank you and another to thank you from the heart. True gratitude is unconditional giving and is not related to any form of agreement or defect, that is. I will be grateful, so I get good things back.

Appreciation is about receiving and flowing love. When you value something, you open your heart and accept the love of the object or person you value. Again, the true understanding is about having an open heart and not about responding to a need or defect.

Strangely enough, people (at least in Western society) are not very good at gratitude or appreciation, although that doesn't mean you can't learn. You might think that there is nothing better than giving and receiving love, and that is true. It's just that you can hang on to issues that have to do with trust and value, and so most expressions of gratitude and appreciation come with general terms and conditions.

How can you change that to be truly grateful and appreciated?

Like many things, the answer lies in the heart and a little straightforward practice and perseverance.When you give gratitude, you offer a connection with love within yourself. You spread the love of the world in one focus - usually to another. Of course, you can love only if you can achieve the love that is in you (and always is whatever happens).

Joining is also the key to recognition, although this time love comes to you and asks to be accepted, and it is your job to let this love enter. As gratitude, you have to open your heart to make it happen.

An open heart and a connection to inner love are therefore essential for gratitude and appreciation. An open heart allows the flow of love without restriction inside and outside. Then try.

Close your eyes and take a deep breath. Every time you retreat, you tell yourself to "let go" and feel that he let go of everything. Then the love that is always in your heart will begin to spread in your body until you feel full. Continue spreading this love until you are surrounded. You can experience it as a deep feeling or a feeling of being filled and surrounded by light. You can feel very connected or just very loving. Whatever you feel, in this state it is natural to give gratitude and gain recognition.

Healthy food for a happy life

A healthy diet is the most important thing for a happy life. Exercise and healthy nutrition are the two most important factors for the growth and maintenance of a healthy body. Being obese increases the risk of diabetes, heart attack, blood pressure, breathing problems, arthritis, osteoarthritis, etc.

Being overweight is a big problem that affects millions of people in the United States. A fifth of the population of American adults is obese.

According to various medical journals, the United States has never been so overweight. Taking the right kind of food helps a lot in maintaining good health.

Eating food that is high in fat and high in carbohydrates is not good for your health. Taking more aerated drinks is very bad for your health. So try to avoid it. Drink plenty of water, soy milk or skimmed milk. Train daily or at least 5 days a week. 30 minutes a day cycling, jogging or any aerobic exercise helps the body relieve stress and maintain a healthy body.

Most people try to take food even when their stomach is full. While they watch TV, play video games, they continue to eat even when their stomach is full. Eat lots of fruits and vegetables every day. Try to avoid pre-packaged food, such as food stored in cans. Never skip breakfast and chew food well so that you have no stomach problems.

The importance of happiness

Happiness can be said to be the elusive feeling that comes and goes that we all long for. Few people know its true meaning because most people simply consider it as a feeling when they have achieved a goal. It is just a given right.

Why is it important that you ask yourself. Even if life is as complicated as it is, you are still part of having a balance of metabolic hormones that control the state of your body that is responsible for your body's well-being. These emotions bring out the positive in you and enable you to tap and use this positive energy to share it with the universe around you.

Many people suffer from such ailments and unfortunate events, while others cannot sustain their families due to a lack of or loss of jobs during the recession. It may be difficult but in all of us the glimpse of the light that forgets everything that may have happened to us looks at the good that we have achieved so far and uses us to lift us out of debt that seems too deep.

It is a well-known, scientific fact that grief is responsible for more underlying diseases and diseases, such as migraines and the like, in society as we know it today. It is no wonder that there are too many prescriptions and the use of many antidepressants to cope with their situations. Such medication is not the cure, it only acts like a pillow and the symptoms continue to manifest.

In recent decades there has been a major development in coaching and therapy. We all know that prevention is better than cure, so it is important to evaluate and value the use of the two.

Training and developing your mind is an important way to make sure that you know how to use that important form of energy, everything you know is good, and gives you memories of past events that can be your determination and determination Strengthen to Overcoming an obstacle can be your way. A life counselor will help you train you in understanding the power of your mind over matter and how you can achieve your goals.

THE CORNERSTONE OF LIFE - EVERY HAPPY LIFE DEPENDS ON A PLANNED BASIS

The cornerstone of your life is the most important, fundamental, essential and essential stable element of your successful future. Therefore, focus your attention on values that have been historically endorsed by religions and cultures, such as loyalty, humility, integrity, courage, generosity, compassion, and perseverance.When you collect ingredients to create the cornerstone of your life, conscious knowledge of your character, motives, desires, and feelings is necessary.

If you know each other well, you can better use your strengths and weaknesses to avoid distractions from people, things, and places that are incompatible with the real ones.Clearly understand your important underlying beliefs and values so you can focus and use your energy to achieve your goals. Understand that glory, power and wealth are not goals that value your most important values.

In the construction of the building, the cornerstone

supports the entire building. When the building is removed, it falls apart. This cornerstone is important because all other bricks are placed regarding this brick and therefore determine the location of the whole structure.

The same principles apply to the cornerstone of life. Your life is a structure. It consists of various complex parts and the arrangement and relationship of parts or elements of your life always create individual complexities.Your attitude and determination to deal with difficult life situations and solve every problem, if any, will prove to be the solution for building your cornerstone in life.If you understand where you want to be, you can run your actions every day to get closer to your goal.Develop your basic plan so that it will be difficult to change character, defeat or spread. Let this plan be your center of operations to focus your thoughts and actions as you develop your cornerstone of life. Let this 'plan' be your assumption and assumption.After all, I am very aware that "happiness" is the necessary element of your plan and the construction of your cornerstone for life.

Happiness is a state of mind or mental state of well-being that is characterized by positive emotions ranging from satisfaction to intense joy. Happiness is a choice that you have to make. It is a state of being that only you can create. Finding real happiness is a very personal journey. It is found during the journey, not the place you visit or stays or stops.

Happiness is a feeling of inner peace and satisfaction. Avoid worry, anxiety, and obsession with thoughts. Stop and meditate every day. It is easier to choose happiness when the mind becomes peaceful.Do not take everyday things in life for granted. Give back a smile with kind words. I appreciate the beauty of God all around you. Be thankful that you are not hungry and be a true friend to your friends.

Lower your lifestyle and enjoy the real quality of life every day. Avoid the disc only to get a number or quantity of something.Understand and believe that you can more easily overcome fear, anxiety, and sadness if you accept them as a natural part of everyone's daily life. This can lead to happiness.

You can more easily enjoy satisfaction and enjoyment at work and home when the things you do are fun. Be committed to your work, work, career, mission and the importance of what you do from the moment you wake up every day.

Your initiative at work can increase your happiness. In other words; Enjoying your work and work is more important than working on a work that you don't like, just putting more money in the bank. Satisfaction, not wealth can make you happy. You can lose your health and not enjoy the money.

The great thing is that happiness can be learned, but you have to learn early in life. For example: as we grow older, we need friends and not dollars. To have friends, we need happy thoughts and happy activities.

Studies have shown that you cannot change your genes or your nature. About 50% of your traits are genetically determined (hereditary) traits or traits.

For example, you can check your weight, but you cannot change it. If you are an extrovert, overly expressive person, mainly concerned with external things or objective considerations, you cannot change this extrovert attribute. If you tend to see the worst aspect of things or think that the worst will happen and you have a lack of hope or confidence in the future, you cannot change this pessimistic trait.Another 50% of your movements come from training and habits. In this positive area, you need to concentrate your strenuous physical or mental efforts to change your behavior and patterns of thought to maximize happiness in every mental and physical cell in your body.

Focus on the positive and avoid the negative! You must fill your mind with happy thoughts that make you want to live and be active with others. Joining charities increases your overall wellbeing. Help neighbors, sign up, donate goods and services, pass on your skills, show forgiveness, and listen to a friend.

Consider a risky or courageous journey or business. You can not expect anything if you never take any risk. "Those who dare don't win anything."

Train today and every day and enjoy the benefits of long-term effects. Exercise reduces depression, gives you a sense of satisfaction, gives you a good feeling, increases self-confidence and gives you a chance to meet people.Maximize your happy thoughts, actions, and current relationships or events. Check every opportunity for happiness. Surround yourself with family and friends and enjoy their friendship. Spend more time with friends. People who have a lot of friends and spend a lot of time with friends are happier. Always remember your family and make new friends.

Train to think about happy thoughts. Be grateful and loving and express these qualities. Always try to smile and express optimism. Say "thank you" and I'm serious. Remember, trying to keep up with Joneses is bad for your trust and happiness.

Research shows that spouses are generally happier than individuals. People who enjoy life are usually happier in their marriage.You need to look around and watch others calmly and attentively at every step of your community. You may be surprised that many or most people with extraordinary talent or people who focus on wealth, beauty, fame and strength are not "happy runners".

Stop by and take the time to "smell the roses". Then try to watch the children playing.You are probably happier when your basic needs (food, water, shelter) are met.People who have a lot of friends and spend a lot of time with friends are happier.Studies show that the following is not related to happiness:

- Race
- Climate
- Level of education
- More money
- Perfect health. (The degree of ill health does not

mean accident, but serious illnesses).

Understand the definition of "assumptions" and "conjectures" and apply them to your life.

When developing a master plan for your "cornerstone of life", consider the following:

- Personal features that you feel others in you.
- Important lessons that you think you have learned in your life.
- Work or pleasure you are satisfied with.
- What brought you the greatest joy today?
- What would you like to see on your tombstone?